A Glass Half Full

Drinking: Reducing the Harm

Andy Stonard

A Glass Half Full

Published in Great Britain in 2012
by Little Dice

Copyright 2012 © Andy Stonard

ISBN 978-0-9562265-4-9

Little Dice
Trinity Farm, Middleton Quernhow
Ripon, North Yorkshire
HG4 5HX
United Kingdom

PART 1

PART 2

PART 3

A Glass Half Full

Introduction

The Sanity of the United Kingdom

I was having a conversation recently with a French friend in deepest rural France. They wanted to practice their English. The conversation turned to drinking in the United Kingdom, because of my work. I had been telling her some facts and figures. She suddenly stopped me speaking by raising a hand.

'So let me repeat what you have been telling me. According to your government's own statistics there are over eight million people drinking over recommended safe levels and you are in the minority if you drink under sensible limits according to another piece of research?'

'Yes', I replied.

'And is it true that according to your drug classifications, alcohol is considered the third most dangerous drug available?'

'Yes'

'That alcohol is involved in 50 per cent of domestic violence and in stranger violence?'

'Yes', I nodded

'Your hospitals have over one quarter of their beds with patients who have alcohol-related ill health and come the evening over 80 per cent of people at Accident and Emergency have been drinking?'

'That's correct.'

'Yet you have over 100,000 licensed premises and retail outlets across the country?'

'Correct again.'

'And your government earns over £14 billion from this misery?'

'Yes'.

'*Sacre Bleu*. I thought it was my English that was bad because I could not believe such madness.'

The statistics quoted above are not taken from an anti-alcohol group or pressure group, they are the governments own statistics. They appeared in a government document entitled 'Alcohol Harm Reduction Strategy for England and Wales'. It was produced by the previous Labour government under Tony Blair.

This strategy was produced through the Cabinet Office and the consultation was widespread and thorough. The people involved in the development who I met were fiercely bright and intelligent, though I would say from my perspective lacking more than a little in humour.

To this day, I wonder whether the title they gave this document did reflect their brightness and masked a wonderful sense of humour.

Sadly, I do not think this was the case.

The Alcohol Harm Reduction Strategy for England and Wales (if you drop the principality) creates the abbreviation AHRSE. For many of us working in the field of alcohol misuse, a better title could not be found.

The findings confirmed everything that most people knew already. The strategic actions came with no money attached to it, no one person, no department to lead on it, no reporting mechanisms and no statutory duties attached to it.

Even worse, it was produced in the same year the government produced a new Licensing Act. This Licensing Act actually increased opening times (and introduced the so called 24 hour licensing arrangement). In fact the Alcohol Strategy was still being consulted on when the Licensing Act was becoming legislation. They had already made up their mind about the direction they wanted to go in, what they wanted in the strategy and more importantly, what they did not want to have in the strategy - so much then, for open consultation and open government.

The then Minister of Health would have us believe (with a straight face) that extended hours without any other change in strategy or thinking about alcohol, would actually lead to a reduction in consumption and alcohol-related disorder because everyone would drink more steadily and not rush to beat last orders.

It is actually very hard to articulate an argument against what the Minister claimed, as this suggestion renders most people incredulous and as a result quite speechless through shock.

Simply overnight, instead of not being served after 11.00 pm in a pub or at midnight or 1.00 in the morning in a club, we could sit there for a further one, two or three hours and not drink anymore. I do not think so. Whatever can be said about the united Kingdom, its people have never had the reputation as a sipping nation when it comes to imbibing alcohol.

However, it is redolent of many government strategies and initiatives – policy is driven not by evidence but by political motivation, sometimes by expediency and in this case wishful and naïve thinking. Is it better than no policy at all? When it comes to alcohol and the track record of the last thirty years then I actually doubt it.

In 2012, not to be outdone, the Coalition government under David Cameron have produced a new Alcohol Strategy. This of course promises a new approach, blames the previous government for most of the problems (which is at least consistent with every other new approach that they have taken).

This is the opening of Prime Minister Cameron's forward to the Strategy:

Binge drinking isn't some fringe issue, it accounts for half of all alcohol consumed in this country. The crime and violence it causes drains resources in our hospitals, generates mayhem on our streets and spreads fear in our communities. My message is simple. We can't go on like this. We have to tackle the scourge of violence caused by binge drinking. And we have to do it now.

This forward is reproduced in the back of this book (I did not want to turn you off the book right at the beginning), but he also goes on to suggest:

This strategy sets out how we will attack it from every angle. More powers to stop serving alcohol to people who are already drunk. More powers for local areas to restrict opening and closing times, control the density of licensed premises and charge a late night levy to support policing. More powers for hospitals not just to tackle the drunks turning up in A&E – but also the problem clubs that send them there night after night. And a real effort to get to grips with the root cause of the problem. And that means coming down hard on cheap alcohol.

When beer is cheaper than water, it's just too easy for people to get drunk on cheap alcohol at home before they even set foot in the pub.

So we are going to introduce a new minimum unit price.

My take on much of this so called new approach is that it is referencing existing legislation with the promise to actually enact it this time. However, the most significant strand of the strategy is based on addressing binge drinking through minimum unit pricing. At one stage he appears to be suggesting that it is based on the premise that we have the situation where beer is cheaper than water and it is this that causes the mayhem in city centres and the crime in our communities. I have to say that this is more than a little concerning. It is not cheap booze that causes mayhem in city centres – it is people. These people are often intoxicated on a mix of drinking at home, in pubs and in clubs (where drinks are far from cheap).

Prime Minister Cameron states that this is no fringe issue. Bloody right this is no fringe issue. The last government Strategy under Prime Minister Blair never claimed that it was a fringe issue either.

This new strategy is about addressing mayhem in city centres and crime in the community, which is the Home Secretary's remit. This is where it becomes scary because it goes to the heart of this book. The Home Secretary, Theresa May, assisted in the launch of this strategy by appearing on BBC Breakfast. Presumably, as one of the leading brains behind this 'new approach' she was sailing along admirably as the concerned Home Secretary coming to our rescue across the seas of drunken crime until she was asked a very simple question:

'How much do you drink in a week? Do you know how many units per week?'

To which the Home Secretary answered:

'I look at what I drink in a week... I enjoy a drink as most people do...'

The interviewer interrupts her:

'The question was very simple – do you know how many units you drink?'

'It varies from week to week.'

'So you don't know?'

The Home Secretary looking more than a little uncomfortable (and I would say irritated):

'I could give you a guess on the number of units I drink each week but as I said I enjoy a drink but I am not someone who causes mayhem in city centres when I drink.'

The notes above from the TV appearance are not word perfect but it is an accurate reflection of the interview. The point of repeating it here is for two reasons. Firstly, most of us do not know how much we drink each week and units of alcohol to most people are an irrelevance when it comes to having a drink, hard to measure and completely the wrong psychology. In that respect, I felt sorry for Theresa May because she answered like most of us do – a little unsure, our intimacy slightly invaded and our mathematical brain not up to the speed of questioning. Secondly, as Home Secretary, leading on a national alcohol strategy aimed at reducing alcohol-related crime it was shameful and inspired absolutely no confidence that one of the main architects of the strategy really understood what she was trying to tell us about how to drink and behave.

Drinking alcohol in Britain has again become a perilous pastime. As you will read in this book, there have been periods in history when the people have drunk more (much more, in fact) and there have been periods of time when it has greatly fallen because of laws or circumstance (the 1914–18 Great War being such a period).

Our overall level of consumption has decreased slightly in recent years, but alcohol-related ill health is climbing alarmingly. There is something therefore seriously wrong here.

This book considers the drinking of alcohol in relation to individual drinking patterns, our behaviour, our culture and our attitudes. We cannot just talk about quantity and arrange our policies and public education around quantity. It is discussing Alcohol UK. How its people consume alcohol. How alcohol relates to ill health, social disorder and violence, child care and domestic violence, our social and moral frameworks are all framed within our drinking and how we drink.

Drinking for some is an occasional pleasure. For many it forms a significant part of their social and personal lifestyle. Then for a large number of people it has become an essential aspect of life where drinking forms an integral daily activity.

For up to two million people it is a daily occupation often from the moment of waking until the end of the day, encompassing psychological and physical dependence. For this group and some of the above, drinking and alcohol-related problems sweep through and affect loved ones and family, neighbours and friends, work colleagues, even strangers on the streets and in the bars.

Then there are those who do not drink, either because they can no longer drink or do not want to drink, those who do not drink because of their religious or spiritual beliefs and those who just do not like the taste or effect of alcohol. Within this group those who can longer drink because they cannot or dare not form a very significant group.

As we shall see later, most of this group consider that they have an individualised illness or condition that means that just one drink will lead to a relapse of the condition or illness of alcoholism. This has become the mainstream approach to alcohol in relation to dependency on alcohol and is also the main theme of Alcoholics Anonymous (AA) – salvation or the chance of a new and better life through abstinence.

This international self-help group is truly effective and the membership is anonymous, is not religious nor is it affiliated to any other group. Neither is it political. It is a massive group of people who choose not use their experiences in any other way but to help both themselves and others to stay abstinent or to find abstinence.

It is a most amazing network and many men and women I know have found comfort and support through these groups and individual members. They are the most impressive self–help group that I know of. My point is that as a group they have the potential to be a truly influential group on the politics and economics of the UK (and around the world) but choose not to. They choose not to because to an individual they consider themselves to be personally responsible for their own situation a self-induced condition, illness or disease, a personal weakness or in the genes or inherited through social conditioning or personality traits.

Such a dynamic is quite remarkable and a very significant component in the overall picture.

Alcohol consumption (as demonstrated in the AHRSE) is a significant factor in domestic violence and child abuse, in violent incidents and in accidents on the roads, in the work place and in the home. The NHS services (especially A & E), GP surgeries, the police service and the courts are often overwhelmed with drunkenness and the accompanying chaos that comes in its wake. We know all this of course. Such statistics appear regularly in our newspapers and in the media

The interesting issue amongst these horrifying statistics is that many of the problems associated with drinking are not always about the amount that is drunk but about the behaviour that occurs as a result of the drinking, whether it is the cause or the convenient vehicle for the behaviour to occur.

Against this reality we have a range of political and economic commentaries on how best to tackle this from the government but with no action and never anything concrete. The drinks industry advertise and promote brands and sell alcoholic beverages very successfully. The supermarkets sell vast amounts of discounted lager and wines as part of their marketing strategies. Local corner shops have to have a licence to sell alcohol or go out of business.

On the opposing side the British Medical Association (BMA) and health lobby, the police and local authorities all caution against the wave of alcohol-related ill health and harm, our hospital services are overrun, whilst whole city centres are drunk with serious disorder and violence, often on the brink of major confrontations and disaster.

This can only be likened to an on-going re-organisation of deck chairs on the Titanic.

The one dominating theme through the last thirty years is that no one from any of these of these 'interests' can find anything to agree on. What they do instead is to regurgitate the same old arguments about raising the price of alcohol which will reduce overall consumption, dispute opening times and argue whether the licensed trade should be restrained through statute and regulation or allowed to continue to tighten up through self-regulation. What this of course does is to penalise the majority for the 'sins' of the minority.

In AA they will often talk about an individual needing to reach their rock bottom (their lowest point) before they can begin to recover. The diagram of this is usually portrayed as descending down a slope into the bottom and an equal slope up the other side. It looks like a gorge.

Collectively, we (the people of the UK) are at the bottom of that gorge. At the top of the gorge, on one side are the drinks industry and trade, with those who argue for freedom of choice and on the other side are those from public health, the moralists and anti–drinks lobbyists. For the last thirty years, they have stood on either side, lobbing accusations and insults, like bricks, at one another. There is no debate, the two sides have their sound bites and their agendas, the bricks just rain down on us below.

What about our politicians? Our Members of Parliament have historically offered nothing coherent and their views and opinions usually divide equally into three. One third will stand on the side of freedom of choice for the consumer and free trade for the industry because it suits them as shareholders, or directors, or as a member of parliament of a constituency with brewing and distilling interests, as donators to party funds, family interests and so forth. Another third will be over with Public Health because of their interests and a third will totally ignore the debate.

Why change the status quo? For the aforementioned combatants, it is a good living working for either side, for the government it is a massive earner and anyway the people of the

UK like a drink and getting drunk. No one forces anyone to drink, we all have free will.

Where do we even try to address such a widespread issue?

Well, my starting point is that I have yet to meet or hear a politician prepared to do anything about it, so we all need to look to ourselves and one another. We need to understand our own attitudes to drinking alcohol, what these attitudes are, how they have been formed and how others' beliefs and attitudes impact on each of us. If your drinking has developed into a 'problem', it is usually a label that has been attached to you by a third party. It is also likely that you already knew that your drinking was a little problematic or needed to be reduced, but accepting it or admitting it is a very different matter. However, it will be individualised and terms like 'lack of will power', 'weakness' and 'it is in the family' will be bandied around. You will not be seen as a victim of advertising and promotion, of governmental acceptance and intransigence.

Basically, everyone is OK until they drink too much or develop the problem – whether it's a teenager admitted to A & E for a stomach pump, to the man who suddenly hits his partner, to someone getting into a fight, to a drunk driver. The first incident is usually labelled out of character, or provocation. It is a shock and is accepted with annoyance but forgiveness. It appears to be a self -induced label, almost a knee jerk reaction to distance ourselves and the person we know from the full blown drunk on the street, the alcoholic who lives down the road.

No one wakes up one morning and decides to have a drink problem, to be an alcoholic. For many it is a slow journey over years. For others it is an unfortunate accident or incident. For some alcohol covers up anxiety, a drink makes socialising easier and for many of us it becomes a daily habit, a bottle of wine at home, a weekend drinking with friends, the pub after work. It builds, it wanes and it builds again.

Holidays involve more drinking, as do weekends because for many they do not have to go to work. You can go shopping at the supermarket and you buy six bottles instead of four because of the discount.

This is all against a background of being told how much or how little we should drink and there lies the rub. Who do you believe? Who can you trust?

One side of the gorge is telling us that you should drink very little to be safe and the other side is offering products that are relatively cheap and enjoyable (and, to be fair, are telling us to be careful when we are enjoying ourselves).

What is this book about?

This book is in three parts – the first part tries to understand how the hell we have come to this situation - culturally, politically, economically and morally. How and why those responsible for alcohol policy have failed us and how our politicians and institutions have abandoned us. How they have reduced the issues and the messages into short term meaningless sound bites.

The reality for most of us is that we are going to have to deal with our personal alcohol problem ourselves or through our family and social network. The public health messages are poor and the services thin on the ground. Having an alcohol problem has always been presented as a problem of the individual, as a weakness. It is never seen as structural.

Therefore, the second part, tries to offer practical tips and advice on what to do ourselves, either as an individual or through friends, family, work and communities, irrespective of the seriousness of the problem. It explores what we can do and our ability to change in this vacuum of abandonment.

The final part considers what needs to change and how this could be done.

The idea is for anyone to pick this book up and hopefully gain a little knowledge about alcohol, drinking and our culture.

This book is designed to consider alcohol from a *harm reduction* perspective – how to enable anyone themselves to reduce the harm, how to be supportive as a parent, partner, relative, friend, lover, colleague; or as a professional.

Harm reduction can ultimately lead to not drinking and being clear that you are now abstinent. However, for many people, simply cutting down on the regularity or amount of drinking, changing attitudes—and therefore behaviour—will start to bring an end to the problem. A little bit of knowledge and insight always helps.

You do not have to be an expert. Nothing in this book is rocket science. It is based on common sense, learnt from others' success and good basic information and knowledge.

This book is designed to gain an insight into the wider issues of drinking, the history of interventions and the politics. In this context then Part Two should be a helpful read for every parent, partner, lover, relative and friend; every alcohol and drug worker, social worker, nurse, doctor, GP, psychologist; for every police officer, probation officer, magistrate, judge; for every teacher, housing worker, pharmacist; for everyone who works in human resources, management, every POLITICIAN and everyone in SOCIAL and HEALTH POLICY.

Obviously, as the author I would say this. However, unless there is a cultural shift across out entire society and its institutions and, most importantly, its people, in our attitudes and beliefs, then all the tampering of pricing policy, licensing and moral panics will continue to be 'like pissing in the wind'.

CHAPTER ONE

HOW THE HELL HAVE WE COME TO THIS?

Britain and alcohol

My one chance of media fame came with the opportunity to be a guest on the BBC Daily Politics programme in March 2008 to discuss the issue of 24 hour licensing and binge drinking. I think I had an audience about 250 people around the country! What I had to say on the programme was that by making licensed premises open for longer hours and increasing all the retail outlets available then drinking was bound to increase within the current culture and attitudes that we all hold.

This evaluation on my behalf was hardly rocket science but was a response to the Health Minister at the time. The Minister actually had the temerity to suggest (as has already been said) that with 24 hour licensing, we would just drink more slowly and that consumption would not increase.

However, both the Minister's assertion and my response missed the point. Trying to talk about changes to opening times is looking at one aspect of drinking alcohol in isolation rather than at the wider picture. Indeed, it could be argued that the banning of smoking indoors has had a more profound effect on attendance and drinking in pubs. This then has had a profound impact on drinking at home and buying our booze in the supermarkets – a story of unintended consequences – but it still misses the point.

Britain has had a heavy drinking culture for at least 5,000 years (and well beyond I would imagine) and a quick run through the history of drinking and the cycle of governmental intervention and encouragement makes illuminating study to the situation we are facing today. The problem is not new but the current and last two governments have followed the tradition of previous ones and learnt nothing from history.

The foundation for today's drinking that will haunt this nation for decades into the future can be easily seen. Despite the rhetoric, no one in government has taken alcohol seriously.

What makes it even worse is that many in government remain ignorant of what they have done. It would be generous of me to say it was often inadvertent. Having faced the arrogance of Ministers and Secretaries for State about their attitude to any of us struggling with trying to work with chronic levels of drinking, I cannot find that generosity as I write this. They have simply done what most families and professionals in the health and social services do: deny it, collude with it or ignore it – it is the usual one third, one third and one third.

Our Health Messages

People in Britain are now genuinely confused about what and how they should be drinking. The recommended safe levels are 21 units for men and 14 for women and we are told that bingeing constitutes over 4 units in one session. That is the equivalent to 2.5 pints of bitter and two pints of stronger lager. After 25 years working with alcohol, I am as confused as everyone else.

The levels of consumption on an average Friday night are probably nearer 15 to 25 units and are also termed bingeing.

The health message we have uses units of alcohol. The recommended safe levels are the same if you are eighteen or sixty-five, eight stone or twenty; in good health or bad; on medication or not, rich or poor. On income support, drinking 21 units a week costs 30 per cent of income, but at £50,000 a year just 3 per cent. Alcoholic strengths on wine and beer vary greatly from product to product and units fail completely to address behaviour and as it is our behaviour that changes when drinking this seems like a fundamental flaw to me.

Drinking under 21 units a week is called **sensible**.

Well excuse me but who wants to be f**king **sensible**?

As drinking, on the whole, is a social event, involving talking, laughing, going out, socialising, then **sensible** is not exactly a term that is going to appeal. When you sit in a pub or bar, you want to be safe but not **sensible** – you've probably spent most of the day at work being sensible.

When you start laughing too loudly because someone has just told you a joke whilst on your first pint, who wants to be reminded to be **sensible**?

So, in addition to being sensible, they also introduced the idea of drinking responsibly. Now responsible retailing and the responsibility of any industry around the safety of their products and compliance with health and safety is one thing, but suggesting to a consumer that they need to do something responsibly is another matter. It is highly preferable to being sensible but it is still a sound bite and relatively meaningless. Very few individuals drink with the intention of being sick, of injuring themselves, of getting into a fight, or of knowingly contract a venereal disease through not practising safe sex.

That is the trouble with sound bites – they come without information and education. They come without understanding and instead are delivered with assumptions.

UNITS OF ALCOHOL

Here is the official guidance on a selection of drinks:

One pint of strong lager (alcohol 5 per cent vol)
= 3 units

One pint of standard strength lager (alcohol 3 - 3.5 per cent vol)
= 2 units

One 275ml bottle of an alcopop (alcohol 5.5 per cent vol)
= 1.5 units

One standard (175ml) glass of wine (alcohol 12 per cent vol)
= 2 units

Easy isn't it? So you are advised to drink no more than 21 units per week if you are a man, so that is one pint of strong lager per day (7 days x 3 units). You are also advised not to binge drink. Bingeing is classified as more than 4 units, which is one pint and a third. Have you ever tried to order a third of a pint? If you have a half on top of that pint then you're officially bingeing.

The smart arse health practitioner would tell you to shift to a lower strength lager or to drink a non-alcoholic beverage but if you get my drift then they are somewhat missing the point.

Then to make it all sound even more far fetched, we label this health message under SENSIBLE DRINKING. It is as much in touch with the reality of life and drinking behaviour as Tony Blair telling us there were weapons of mass destruction in Iraq.

To make matters worse the alcoholic products keep changing in strength. Most of our wines are now nearly twice as strong as they were ten years ago. Our lagers and beers are all different to one another.

These recommended safe drinking levels were clearly explained in the AHRSE (Alcohol Harm Reduction Strategy for England and Wales). These have not changed with the 2012 government Alcohol Strategy. Indeed when you go through all the key documents of the last 20 years from *Calling Time* in 2000 back to the Lord President's *Report on Alcohol Misuse* in 1991, you will find reference to units. In 1987 the Royal Colleges confirmed their support for safe drinking limits measured in units of alcohol.

This was because in the 1980s there was plenty of research from 'liver experts' on the organ's ability to process various products, including alcohol. Parallel to this, there was the debate on legal drink driving limits and safe drink driving limits (notice the discrepancy), neither of which have any relation to sensible drinking levels. A sensible day's consumption will take you over the legal drink driving limit and that is not very sensible either is it?

As an aside, I was 'lucky enough' to attend the 2nd International Conference on Alcohol and Harm Reduction in 2005 in which the then Russian definition of a drink driving offence is 'displaying drunkenness'. So not all the world is in harmony with units and what constitutes safe drink driving.

You can read all of this research on the Net (if you really do have the time or the inclination). However, all the research is by a group of highly qualified and esteemed doctors and researchers who talk of units of alcohol, average processing times by the liver and what constitutes sensible drinking levels.

Welcome to the world of UNITS OF ALCOHOL and SENSIBLE DRINKING LIMITS.

What did these bastions of SENSIBLE DRINKING HABITS have in common?

All highly qualified in their fields.

All medically trained.
All from Social Class 1 or 2.

In other words, nearly all of them were well paid and middle aged. They were almost exclusively white men, all having trod the well worn path of medical training. This is what usually lays the path of Public Health for the masses designed by the exclusive few.

However, if you go back on the Net with me you will find plenty of research that states that sex, age, and weight all have a significant impact on the ability of the body and the liver to function with alcohol and to process the alcohol. Some of it is as simple as basic maths. Yet show me the evidence that our Public Health Consultants ever factored this in.

So, in effect, anyone between the age of 18 and 80, an eight stone jockey through to a Sumo Wrestler can drink the same sensible amounts and be safe. An 18 year old teenager can drink the same amount as an Octogenarian! Well that's just plain rubbish.

So sex, age and weight all have an influence. What else does?

How about medication?
How about diets?
How about health?
What about pregnancy?

Yes of course they all have an influence and there is reference to all these in NHS publications and research.

Now what about Ethnicity/Culture/Spiritual Beliefs?

There is again plenty of research on alcohol and its effects on behaviour on different ethnic groups. Certain communities are physically more susceptible to alcohol than others. Research on indigenous groups and the impact of alcohol such as the aboriginal peoples is fairly clear cut.

I've spent the last 25 years living in north London. The communities who make up that part of London are indeed diverse and different. They come from a range of ethnic, religious, spiritual and political backgrounds. For some of those groups, abstinence from alcohol is the norm; for others it is tolerated, whilst for others, alcohol performs certain roles in particular functions or ceremonies.

For others alcohol is part of the fabric of everyday life. Younger generations who grow up in such a multi-racial setting drink in defiance of, or as part of, a cultural mesh with peers.

That is sufficient evidence for me to believe that the blanket approach of UNITS is simply not good enough.

Now, what about alcohol and class?
What about alcohol and income?

The table below is a rough attempt to demonstrate the effect of expenditure on alcohol, against income. £5,000 is income support plus a few extras; a state pension or thereabouts.

Units per week	Income	Income	Income
	£5,000	**£15,000**	**£50,000**
21-28 (£30 per week)	£1,560 (30%)	£1,560 (10%)	£1,560 (3%)
30-50 (£45 per week)	£2,340 (40%)	£2,340 (15%)	£2,340 (6%)
Over 70 (£60 per week)	£3,120 (60%)	£3,120 (20%)	£3,120 (7%)

On £5,000 per year, if you drink within sensible drinking limits you will spend 30 per cent of your income, which is not sensible. If you earn £50,000 a year and drink within sensible drinking limits you will spend three per cent of your income, which is very sensible.

It is not unreasonable to enjoy a modicum of sensible drinking whatever your income, but on £5,000 a year to even drink sensibly as the experts tell you, you have to make cut backs on other essentials such as food, heating and clothing. It is good old supply and demand economics.

Put simply, the richer you are, the less impact alcohol has on your lifestyle barring accidents or an existing health problem. Now that is the 'bleeding obvious'. However, if I was to cite Alcohol Concern's statistics and say that 80 per cent of alcohol-related ill health occurs in the poorest 10 per cent of the population then that table makes compelling reading. It is all part of the poverty trap. Are all people on low incomes therefore compelled to not drink?

Certainly the drinks industry and the government do not want them to stop and public health messages make no reference to drinking even more sensibly (or abstaining) if you are poor.

Winston Churchill, it is alleged, consumed something like a bottle of brandy and champagne a day during the war. Whether this is true or not, he certainly did a pretty good job and, anyway, who could blame him for drinking with such a stressful job. I doubt he worried about his units.

The Queen Mother was another person who many commentators have suggested liked a drink and it never did her any harm. Whether this was true, she was on a pretty good income, in heated accommodation and probably never had to wash her own underwear. She did not have to worry about units and lived a long and happy life.

We have to make up our minds what we are saying. On the one hand I am told that alcohol has no respect for class. Alcoholism is an illness or disease that can strike down any one of us if we stray from the path. It is this message that is encompassed in UNITS. That's why we should all be SENSIBLE.

But UNITS of SENSIBLE drinking are only OK as long as you ignore all of the following:

Sex
Age
Weight
Medication

Diet
Ethnicity/Culture/Class
Income
Environment

So, what is the alternative for addressing drinking alcohol?

Behaviour

Drinking alcohol affects how we behave. Alcohol, to quote a favourite line from our esteemed medical profession, is "Britain's favourite drug". It is a powerful substance that affects cognition immediately. It affects emotion, motor control, judgement and more.

The process takes effect in a reasonably steady way. How we choose to use the drug and behave under its increasing effect is the key. Understanding how we behave and think under the influence of alcohol, how we choose to use alcohol and to justify our behaviour is an individual choice. It comes from a mixture of learnt behaviour, education and the information we are given. This is the basis for my colleagues' therapeutic work. Why, I ask, is it different as a health message?

Alcohol and accidents; alcohol and aggression, alcohol and violence are the reality partnerships. You avoid all of these if you live by the SENSIBLE drinking message.

It is not true. Statistically speaking, SENSIBLE drinking puts you in the frame for alcohol-related accidents, being a victim of crime, domestic and stranger violence. It does not matter how rich you are, you are in the frame.

The reality is that no one really wants to be sensible. Even if you are going down the pub for an orange juice, you want to relax, to talk and socialise, to laugh, to enjoy friendship and company. You want to be safe but not sensible. Sensible is a good word but it is loaded. Being sensible usually has connotations of behaving on someone else's terms, being cautious, holding back in some way, behaving in some way that is not necessarily the usual.

If we are to teach about drinking then we need to talk about how to self-assess risk. To be able to self-assess risk, firstly you need good basic information that is not loaded—not messages but information.

You need to make people understand how their brain works and how its functioning is altered under the influence of a drug. You need to make people understand that there is no 'one size fits all' solution such as units, and that quantity or volume is only one viewpoint. Looked at in isolation it can be completely misleading.

Weekends in city centres for many are about 'getting smashed', often before they even go out. It is about attitude and subsequent behaviour. The pubs and clubs are not promoting sensible drinking because they have a business to run and they have staff to cope with those who become drunk or misbehave. So long as they quell disorder on their premises it is no longer their problem when their customers are ejected into the streets.

A & E and the police are swamped with drunkenness, city centres become no go areas for people over thirty and the newspapers and TV run shock programmes and articles on slow news weeks.

To be fair, Diageo have paid for a series of adverts on this – they are well produced, expensive and appropriate adverts, but they are geared to an audience on TV that is not in the pub or club or under the influence. Similarly, you can pick up a leaflet in a GP surgery or library but not in a pub or club or at the till of a supermarket or off-licence.

After a couple of drinks, I swear I look a little thinner and have more hair on the top of my head. Aches and pains recede. I'm no different to anyone else in the room.

Drinking is like going through a time tunnel. At every stage the likelihood of certain thoughts, events and the possibility of incidents are all there.

You may have come to the conclusion, that as a worker in the field of alcohol use and misuse, I do not like UNITS. I also do not like them as a consumer. For starters, the entire message has me obsessed about intake rather than behaviour. One night a week at least I am labelled as a binger; some weeks I am a very SENSIBLE drinker and other weeks, because of a birthday or friends staying, I am a HEAVY or at RISK drinker.

It's no different to the plethora of concerns I and friends and relatives have about high and low blood pressure monitoring, cholesterol levels, diets, and addictive behaviours ranging from shopping and gambling through to sex and cosmetic surgery. The anxiety is usually in the message—or not understanding the message—especially in relation to your own lifestyle, feelings and concerns.

My frustration with health zealots and their messages reached its zenith at the same conference I referred to earlier about the Russian definition of drink driving.

An American health campaigner, having dismissed with disdain the Russians, referred to her campaign for safer driving in Bangalore and parts of Eastern Europe, as lives touched by her and her colleagues, in her head count of clients. What she meant to say was that she and her colleagues had distributed 25,000 leaflets through clubs and bars at the end of the night.

In closing I want to take you back to our two most recent alcohol strategies. The Alcohol Harm Reduction Strategy for England and Wales (AHRSE) states that there are over 8 million of us drinking over 28 units per week.

The 2012 government Alcohol Strategy details this in the following way:

We estimate that in a community of 100,000 people, each year:

- *2,000 people will be admitted to hospital with an alcohol-related condition;*

- *1,000 people will be a victim of alcohol-related violent crime;*

- *Over 400 11-15 year olds will be drinking weekly;*

- *Over 13,000 people will binge-drink;*

- *Over 21,500 people will be regularly drinking above the lower-risk levels;*

- *Over 3,000 will be showing some signs of alcohol dependence; and*

- *Over 500 will be moderately or severely dependent on alcohol.*

How we get our health and behaviour information over on drinking and safety is in need of a fundamental review and overhaul. It takes a special kind of health initiative to fail so miserably with so many for so long and for the 'cream' of our medical profession to uphold this failure and stifle debate so effectively.

However, do not mistake this diatribe as an excuse for not underlining the seriousness of the alcohol problem/epidemic that has swept through our society. Young people are dying of liver cirrhosis and alcohol-related accidents and this should not be happening. People are scarred for life and attacked because of people drinking too much and alcohol-related violence.

Our Accident and Emergency clinics are like the Alamo besieged by drunken injuries – all this caused by an attitude towards a legal substance. As this book explains, blaming just the alcohol industry and a few idiots who drink too much is a cheap, shoddy and wholly inaccurate way to describe and address the problem.

Having a whole campaign based on a price hike is a complete failure of a group of highly educated minds (who we have all paid for their education through taxation) who should know better, alongside a government who need to pull out the fence posts from their backsides and be honest – either it's a legal substance from which we earn an absolute fortune and we do not intend to do a thing about it **or** it's a very dangerous drug and is something we need to address in a fundamentally different way.

The middle way of 'tough talking and tough inaction' is the current and previous governments' approach and is best translated as 'it is a legal substance from which we earn an absolute fortune but we really do try to cover this fact up with concentrating on the war on drugs instead and sound as if we are trying to regulate the worst excesses of the market, while in all reality we are doing bugger all….but the deck chairs do look much more effective laid out this way than before!!!'

Economic Relationships

To an observer over the last 30 years, the main argument has appeared to rage between the drinks producers and retailers and the health and alcohol interest lobby. The fundamental component that is constantly ignored is the protagonist – the Treasury.

The relationship between the treasury and alcohol is a fundamental issue that needs to be properly explored and never is. With an income of around £14 billion from tax and duty (never mind company taxation), successive governments have tried to dress up tax increases as a type of harm reduction on overall consumption.

The fact is that simple economics mean that someone who is physically or psychologically addicted to alcohol will have to find the additional money to maintain the 'habit'. They will do this through sacrificing other things such as food and heating, or on their family.

Any government is always going to be reluctant to deliver the needed reforms to reduce the harm when it will dramatically reduce its income. During the recent recession this £14 billion was a difference between the country being bankrupt and surviving.

Successive British governments have had a sadomasochistic, dependent relationship with alcohol and those who make it and sell it. It is like a doomed and dysfunctional marriage in which neither party can ever contemplate divorce. Dependent on the income, it is tolerant of disorder in city centres and a massive amount of alcohol-related crime and violence. The relationship is a macro version of alcohol-related domestic violence in the home.

Some in the drinks industry have produced an economic model for the social harm their products produce and would be prepared to work more closely with the problem, but still argue that it is the Treasury who have the income and choose not to spend it on a reduction of alcohol-related harm

That is why raising the duty and tax on alcohol coupled with shambolic 'get tough' messages is always going to be favoured by successive chancellors.

Regeneration

The regeneration of our city centres involved the creation of shopping malls and the conversion of banks, cinemas and even churches into huge bars and clubs, many with limited seating in order to encourage vertical drinking, which usually means faster consumption. Local authorities had no powers to dictate how few or many licensed premises they could have. Neither is there much evidence that our good burghers of local democracy were too troubled on allowing many of these developments to go through planning. Indeed in some city centres these establishments can be next to each other or in a line or cluster along a street or small area. This happened despite there being a wealth of research and reports from around the world that where this happens you get a concentration of people and a concentration of trouble.

But never mind, this was about regenerating city centres and of course bringing in much needed revenue to local authorities and creating jobs (especially for people from Eastern Europe who were prepared to travel for low paid work!). So everyone is a winner – big venues, cheap labour and increased revenue for everyone – drinks all round???!!!???

This had the effect of bringing huge numbers of young people into city centres to drink excessive amounts and then being discharged at roughly the same time to descend on the three burger bars and one taxi rank. No one to this date has ever been charged with serving alcohol to someone who is intoxicated (under existing statute) but it allowed the police to have to dedicate almost their entire workforce on most nights to policing these areas.

This had the effect of older people and families ceasing to go out to restaurants and avoiding the city centres at night like the plague. As more and more bars opened (which was easy to do), the competition brought in more and more drink promotions, which went from happy hour to happy week.

The Licensing Act

The Licensing Act introduced extended licensing hours and a host of other de-regulatory measures which made it harder for local authorities to control their licensed premises despite wording that alluded to the contrary. Unfortunately it was produced at a time when the government was supposed to be working on a national Alcohol Strategy. That Strategy came out afterwards and appeared almost as an afterthought, which with hindsight is exactly what it has proved to be.

The Licensing Act was often referred to as as 24 Hour Licensing, which is what technically it was, but the government Ministers at the time tries to suggest that this was a good thing and would reduce harmful bingeing as people would have longer to drink and not rush their drinks at the end of the evening.

You can appeal against premises being granted a licence but it is insufficient to argue that a tenth, twelve or twentieth pub or nightclub in a city centre is one too many. You can cite that a 100 per cent increase in licensed premises appears to have led to a 100 per cent increase in alcohol-related violence and disorder but it will not stop the licence being granted.

This sought of nonsensical thinking now leaves us with more people drinking more alcohol for longer, as was predicted.

The National Alcohol Strategy

The Alcohol Harm Reduction Strategy for England and Wales was the first national alcohol strategy any government has produced that was all encompassing in what it reported about the scale of the problem.

Unfortunately, it reminds me of a wonderful quote that was given to me at a lecture many years ago:

What's the difference between knowledge and wisdom?

Knowledge is knowing that a tomato is a fruit
Wisdom is not putting a tomato in a fruit salad.

The most shocking parts of the document were the staggering statistics about how serious the problem was. Many of us knew this but it had never appeared all in one place and in a government publication. What was truly unbelievable was that this could be written and published with few, if any, targets, no cash attached to it and no regulatory or statutory responsibilities for it. There was no one to lead on it from the government. No department or specialist unit (such as the National Treatment Agency for Drug Misuse) was allocated to lead it on the ground.

Once it was published, the Cabinet Office appeared to consider its work completed. In the Department of Health there was a small alcohol team but they were given no responsibility for the strategy. There did not appear to be any civil servants, not even in the Home Office or Ministry of Health, who had any responsibility for the strategy. Across all government departments, if anyone was given responsibility in their brief then it appeared to be a priority just below 'political links with New Zealand' or the equivalent.

This was made very evident when, in 2006, £100,000 was made available to every Primary Care Trust (PCT) in the country to spend on alcohol initiatives. In London, only two of the thirty two PCT's actually spent it on alcohol projects.

By the end of the last Labour government in 2010, none of the proposals in the strategy had been taken forward. It was a monumental waste of time and money.

To this day, what I struggle with is the question of why they chose to call it a strategy rather than a report, as the one thing that it was completely devoid of any strategic thought.

It would have been better to write the report with the statistics and one page afterwards with:

And we do not intend to do anything about it.

To be fair to the Coalition government under Prime Minister Cameron, the 2012 Alcohol Strategy *is* a strategy. Whether it is the right strategy only time will tell. In the context of this book, it is proposing to hurtle down all the wrong roads.

The National Drug Strategy

The Labour government chose to exclude our favourite drug (alcohol) from their National Drugs Strategy, which evolved over ten years, despite evidence that 80 per cent of drug users drink over the safe recommended levels and the fact that there were then around 250,000 heavy drug users compared with around 2,500,000 heavy to dependent drinkers, with 8.6 million of us drinking over recommended safe drinking levels (although the alcohol strategy had not been produced when the National Drugs Strategy was created, everyone knew the level of alcohol consumption and related problems).

I once met Keith Halliwell, the so called Drug Czar, who told me he would be foolish to ignore alcohol in the drugs strategy. Well, to cut a long story short, nothing happened on his watch but far be it from me to accuse him of being foolish. Perhaps he argued vociferously behind the scenes for alcohol to be taken seriously.

In stark contrast, the new Drug Strategy states:

This strategy sets out the government's approach to tackling drugs and addressing alcohol dependence.

This will be no easy task because over the last ten years, in everyone's haste to collect the new drugs money, the majority of senior management across Health, the Voluntary Sector, the Home Office, Housing and local authorities quietly concentrated on drugs and abandoned alcohol through neglect – they colluded, ignored or denied it. They pretended that they would do something but none of them did. They would say that they were too busy with the massive changes to drugs.

My question to them is that in this world, when you are at sea in a ship in a storm – do you ignore the people floundering and drowning in the sea? The answer, I am afraid to say was 'yes' from most of my colleagues in the drugs field. One of the really upsetting repercussions of this was that alcohol users were written down as primary drug users if they had a secondary drug problem, especially if this was the only way of accessing any form of treatment. This was widespread and of course skewed the statistics, bringing up the drug numbers and reducing the alcohol numbers who needed treatment.

What the Drug Strategy created was commissioning of new drug services on a massive scale. This commissioning process increasingly re-shaped the existing treatment services in how they wanted it delivered. Many existing treatment models which had been working but were weak through lack of funding, were radically re-organised. The new so called models of care were focussed on criminal justice interventions, massive increases in substitute prescribing and community based services rather than residential treatment.

These types of treatment were not available to those with alcohol misuse problems, nor were they appropriate, but they were the new 'Emperor's clothing' and had not been tested over time, so they were the new way.

Much of the pioneering and successful work within alcohol treatment were working with a model called the cycle of change, with brief interventions, the idea of controlled drinking and relapse prevention (backed up through cognitive behavioural treatment). The brave new drugs world and commissioning structures little understood this and, in truth, cared little for it as it did not produce the kind of outcomes that the drugs monitoring required.

Worse was to follow. The whole way the local authority commissioning processes worked was to create bigger and merged tenders that favoured a small number of ever expanding drug providers (who still claimed to be charities). These organisations could suddenly employ tender teams and the smaller more traditional charities just could not compete.

In terms of economics, the smaller charities could not offer the same value for money that the larger treatment providers claimed that they could. In a matter of years, alcohol services either disappeared or became tucked into the drug treatment contracts and organisations, with their drug strategy and treatment culture.

It became not uncommon for sympathetic drug workers to report that some clients' minor drug use was their main problem in order for them to obtain treatment because if alcohol was their main presenting problem, then they could not receive treatment. This was appalling enough, without the fact that national statistics were being manipulated. They were being manipulated because many of the commissioners asked for this to happen as soon as it became obvious that there was more money being made available if the statistics were better.

Individualising the problem

Alcohol Misuse is seen as an individual problem. Where it ceases to be an individual addiction or weakness and where it is a national and structural problem goes to the heart of this debate and again needs to be explored.

What has happened in the wake of the growing concern about alcohol misuse is the individual being blamed. Tim Martin, the Chief Executive of Wetherspoons, blames media stars; others blame the drinks industry. Our sports stars often appear in the media for their drunken antics yet sport is heavily sponsored by drinks companies.

Indeed, if public figures step out of line with their drinking then it is deeply personalised and is usually presented as personal weakness and 'pressures of the job'

Politicians who experience problems with alcohol are usually colluded with and the problem is denied, until their cover is blown and then they are respectably individualised and eased out of office. It happens to leaders of the opposition parties and it happens to Cabinet Ministers.

Interestingly, with many media stars across film and music, the attention always focuses on drug use, when in moments of careful reflection (usually in their autobiographies or on TV chat shows), they will acknowledge that it was the drinking that caused the problems (and sometimes death). There is sadly a long list of such 'celebrities' who are classic examples of this.

My colleagues and myself have stood almost as observers watching a disaster unfold concerning alcohol over the last 25 years and it will take a brave politician to stand up and admit the mistakes of the past, never mind open up the problem of alcohol misuse to scrutiny and be prepared to move strategically rather than in the term of one parliament.

Public health, alcohol, tobacco and drugs

Alcohol and tobacco are legal substances, drugs are either illegal (whatever their classification) or are prescribed medically. Government policy and Public Health approach all three as separate problems and totally disregard the fact that probably between a third and half us in the UK use at least two of the three.

Tobacco is heavily taxed, banned in public places and indoors, cannot be advertised and is now being placed under the counter with no packaging. The public health programmes are all about cessation and commercially there are a range of nicotine products all marketed as helping people to stop smoking.

Other alternatives to smoking cigarettes are either banned in the UK and most of Europe (such as Snus – which is legal in Sweden and, interestingly enough, Sweden has the lowest lung cancer rates in the whole of Europe), or are available but are not endorsed by Public Health (the electronic cigarettes). This is all really very helpful to the 25 per cent of smokers who appear unable to stop smoking.

Drugs are illegal and a huge amount of money has been made available for treatment. Successive governments have supported the international 'War on Drugs', yet most of the harms are associated with the illegality of the substances, the crime and the deprivation that stems from all of this. Even tinkering around at the edges of reclassification or decriminalisation usually signals the end of a political or professional career and reputation.

Alcohol – well as this book describes, nothing happens except a lot of talking. But when our experts discuss unit pricing do they stop to consider the effect on market forces for cannabis, crack or heroin? I have not heard one consideration. When they drive tobacco further underground do they consider what is happening in the illegal tobacco market, or homegrown cannabis, or the encouragement of organised crime? I see little evidence.

How short are the memories that the platform for organised crime in the USA was alcohol prohibition and yet they are now doing the same for drugs (and no, I am not arguing for the legalisation of drugs but I am saying we need to completely re-evaluate what we are all doing).

On the subject of all three substances, what everyone is consistent on doing is moralising about drugs, alcohol and tobacco. It staggers me how pompous and high minded some people are about smoking, especially as how close we are to having safer products, smokeless tobacco and the ability to smoke less.

Where some groups and communities really struggle about stopping, the middle classes and their educated public health and politicians create an environment where rational debate ceases to be able to be had. We therefore cannot have smoking harm reduction, despite the fact that millions of people could probably cut down significantly if given the help. Instead from the government and the NHS we have smoking cessation and nothing else and a plethora of nicotine replacement products (as long as they are described as a medical replacement product).

Drugs are similar. Drug use and misuse has swept through our cities and shires. It has devastated at least part of a generation. There was an awkward acceptance of treatments like substitute prescribing, needle exchange.

People should stop taking drugs and they should stop smoking but with drinking, people should be more responsible and drink sensibly. Predictably, the harm reduction approaches in drug treatment are on the wane because of pressure from a sectional but influential segment of society.

Climbing out of the Silos

Nature abhors a vacuum – increasing the price on alcohol and tobacco has a number of effects. It should effect overall consumption by bringing it down (we are told), but it also increases the market for illegal imports. The flow of cheap cigarettes from places like the Ukraine is in direct relation to the pricing structures in each country. This is the first response, with the counterfeit cigarettes to follow and their horrendous health implications because of what goes into them. In alcohol, it is the same – illegal importation followed by home brewing and illegal production. It is the latter that kills thousand around the world on a regular basis.

Our health experts appear to little understand economics and markets. Pricing makes us all switch products – you see it in the illegal drug markets and you see it in the NHS with legal medication. You see it across substances. No one considers what raising the unit price of alcohol will have on the cannabis, cocaine and opiate markets.

Evidence and experience appear to point us in the direction that human beings, throughout history and across cultures appear to enjoy the use of substances for a whole host of reasons. How this is done with the minimum of harm and the maximum of enjoyment would appear to be the fundamental solution. Trying to achieve this by looking into individual silos is not the solution.

So part of the solution to alcohol misuse across our society is for this government and its Public Health gurus to earn their highly paid salaries and address the facts, fictions, preconceptions, research and public concerns about alcohol, tobacco and drugs within one coherent policy, with information and messages that we all understand.

An example for me to quote was the arrival of one Arsene Wenger and the transformation of Arsenal football club. Prior to his arrival it was a successful football club but could be performing better. It had a culture of not just heavy drinking but drinking (and some drug taking) that was on a highly destructive level, involving not just drink driving but individuals involved in court cases that were drink related, even imprisonment. Without being there, what I saw was an alternative lifestyle being offered by the new management that did not come out and criticise (when it was justified to do so) but offered extended careers, better performance and enhanced personal attributes. There was no Arsenal alcohol policy or code of conduct but positive change that assisted individuals and then with it the club improved and went on to win the league Championship.

In a nutshell

So, in a nutshell, we have a situation, where it could be considered that is not normal (in the majority) to drink within recommended safe limits, as a result of a failing and inarticulate health measure.

We have a situation in which it is normal to drink standing up in city centre premises which have been regenerated through creating almost industrial sized warehouse drinking establishments, with unrestricted drinking hours, with the resulting fall out of drunkenness, disorder, public nuisance and injury. We have created a situation where it is accepted that the police, local authorities and NHS services can barely cope with the subsequent results.

Meanwhile the Treasury coins in some £14 billion which makes the drug cartels of Escobar *et al.* look distinctly amateur because this money is made wholly legally and yet they are not implicated and do not get the blame.

In the midst of all this, if you raise your head and admit to having an alcohol problem, you are seen as a weak and addicted individual in need of salvation and redemption, whose fate is forever to be an addict in waiting, held in abeyance by abstinence because you will always be one drink away from oblivion.

Oh, and you need to join up to one of the most successful self-help organisations but you have to be anonymous. As a group you cannot have political views or lobby.

Well, fuck me sideways – if you were writing a novel, you wouldn't dare make it up would you?

CHAPTER TWO

A VERY BRIEF HISTORY OF ALCOHOL AND BRITAIN

Drinking alcohol, its social and cultural functions, its journey into being part of our lifestyle and the need to control its consumption are important to understand when we look at drinking today.

Throughout history, the income alcohol has generated for the Treasury of State, Kings and Queens and more latterly Parliament, also help us to understand the double edged sword that alcohol brings to all aspects of society.

Indeed, it has been proposed that the 'English pub' could well have been a major reason why for the last three hundred years there has never been revolution unlike on the Continent. Who knows whether this could be true, but it is an opinion worthy of consideration.

Even in Neolithic times people drank alcohol by fermenting fruit. There are references to drinking alcohol across all ancient texts since then.

Two thousand years ago, our ancestors fermented barley, honey and apples to make 'ale' (beer), mead and cider respectively. The Romans introduced the vine to produce wine and one of the first records of state intervention around harm reduction was a decree in AD 81 by Emperor Domitian to destroy half the vineyards and forbid any more to be planted without Imperial Licence. This was destined to stay in force for over 200 years, as Linsey Kahn recounts:

The vine edict of Domitian in 92, which directed the interests of Italian wine growers, banned the planting of any new vineyards and ordered "half the vineyards in Asia Minor and other provinces to be uprooted" in Roman provinces. The edict was created because of a strong outbreak of famine in the Empire and was designed to increase the production of corn in the Roman Empire by eliminating "mediocre vines occupying land that could be ploughed and was better suited for corn crops than wine-growing.[1]

The taking of strong ale for men fighting in battle, when they were locked in long, arduous and bloody shield walls against one another was recorded in the early centuries.

Drinking and fires were named in the twelfth century as being 'the only plagues in London'. The Ale House ruled and there was widespread drunkenness. The ale was prepared mostly by monks (in AD 569, the Synod announced that drunken priests had to do fifteen days penance for their drunkenness) and the Archbishop of Canterbury actually managed to force some of these ale houses to be closed down.

It was not until 1494 and 1552 that any legislation appeared concerning the licensing of these premises, with drinking to excess being referred to as 'guzzling'. In 1606, an Act of Parliament imposed a fine of five shillings for drunkenness (or six hours in the stocks – could this be old style tagging?).

In order to reduce the import of foreign brandy, the government encouraged the increased manufacture of gin which is made from corn. This encouragement proved a massive success and production soared. It reduced demand for foreign brandy, and gin became so popular that it overtook beer in popularity. Britain subsequently sank into increased drunkenness. The famous painting by Hogarth of 'Gin Lane' sums up the situation. The death rate actually started to exceed the birth rate and the doctors of the time blamed it on the gin.

---

[1] http://www.winelawonreserve.com/2011/08/09/domitians-vine-edict-story-wine-law/

The squalor that most town- and city-dwellers lived in was not commented on. What is important to recognise however, is that it was safer to drink the beer and gin than the water and this was to remain the case until at least the 1930s.

In 1729, the government placed an extra five shillings tax on a gallon of gin, with the preamble to the Act reading:

...the drinking of spirits and strong waters is becoming very common amongst people of inferior rank and the constant and excessive use thereof tends greatly to the destruction of their health, enervating them, and debauching their morals, and driving them into all manner of vice and wickedness.

Subsequent Acts in 1743 and 1751 raised prices further in an attempt to curtail sales. All this did indeed have an impact on consumption. Some historians have suggested that the introduction of tea drinking had an impact on gin consumption – 'tea used by the meanest families, even of the labouring people' contributed to the decline in gin drinking in this period.

Slowly, gin production and consumption started to increase again, then it escalated massively. Britain did not like its more sober state. This increase was alarming. So alarming that in 1830, the Duke of Wellington introduced the Beerhouse Act.

The rationale behind the Beerhouse Act was to try to promote beer as a cheap competitor to gin. The Act abolished the Beer Tax and permitted anyone to sell beer after being given a licence. There was no reference to gin supply; no reference to pricing, no outlets was mentioned. The impact was massive. Literally thousands of beer houses opened everywhere.

At this time, it should be remembered that housing was not only in desperately short supply, but what was available was on the whole in disrepair. It was estimated that 10 per cent of the population lived in cellars; there was massive overcrowding and a huge homeless population.

The staple diet was bread and this was expensive, whilst gin and beer were cheap. In addition, beer and gin were sold in premises that were usually a vast improvement on their 'home'. They were also open for long hours.

The Beerhouse Act did not appear to consider the fact that beer was an intoxicant. The result was that consumption of beer rocketed, but consumption of gin did not radically decline. The response of those who sold gin was to upgrade their premises into what came to be known as Gin Palaces. England could hardly move for alcohol establishments.

A quote at the time sums it all up:

'Everybody is drunk. Those who are not singing are sprawling. The sovereign people are in a beastly state'
　　　　　　　—Sydney Smith, a clergyman and writer

In 1832, the English Temperance movement entered the ring!

Their opening salvo was to abstain from hard liquor (possibly one thinks to curry favour with the Duke), which proved to be a futile gesture. Hence, enter the 'Preston Seven' (who referred to themselves as the seven men of Preston) led by Joseph Livesey (1794–1884) with the pledge of:

'We agree to abstain from all liqueurs of an intoxicating quality, whether ale, porter, wine or ardent spirits, except as medicine.'

(It was not recorded whether the Preston Seven were often ill and in need of medicine!)

Joseph Livesey was regarded as a great social reformer, who was brought up in poverty and squalor. He was the archetypal self-made man, though it is claimed that he never forgot his background. With his new found wealth, he ran his own newspaper and actively campaigned against the Enclosure Act, the Corn Laws and what he considered to be the barbarities of the Poor Law.

At the height of his campaigning and with alcohol consumption extremely high, he wrote in 1862:

'That drink is the source of, the immediate cause of crime, pauperism, disease and insanity'

Strong stuff indeed, eh?
The Temperance movement went on the offensive on two fronts:

The individualistic, personal, moral front.
The legislative and political front.

What they did was to lay the foundation for the dynamics we face today – that alcoholism was a problem of personal responsibility, guilt and self-determinism and that the only way to overcome it was abstinence. It was an individual problem, a moral weakness and the use of alcohol was the root cause of an individual's problems. The only escape was not to drink as there was no other cure. It could only be held in abeyance by not succumbing to the evil substance.

From the original Temperance movement came a proliferation of groups within the movement. These ranged from local Temperance societies, the Order of Good Templars and the Juvenile Templars, the United Kingdom Alliance, the British Women's Temperance Association, the Temperance Friendly Society, the Independent Order of Rechabites, and even the United Kingdom General and Temperance Provident Assurance Company.

Not unnaturally, with such vociferous support, state control of the drink traffic increased. This was the time of the Victorians. Free trade in beer ended in the late 1860s whilst the rise in spirit drinking was finally checked following new licensing legislation in 1872. By 1899, the Report of the Royal Commission on Licensing Laws had bought all trade in intoxicants strictly under the control of the magistrates.

However, the fact remained that by 1913, convictions for drunkenness were still running at 190,000 per year (interestingly enough it is really difficult to access clear and concise current figures on drunkenness arrests/cautions and the other offences/cautions that are given out).

What saved the day for rampant drinking was the onset of the First World War. The slaughter in France had begun. Lloyd George regarded drink as 'the greatest of the three deadly foes – Germany, Austria and drink'. Unfortunately for Britain, not enough Germans were being slaughtered and the production of munitions (especially shells) needed to be stepped up dramatically and done so safely.

To achieve this, the workforce needed to be more productive. To be more productive, they needed to go to bed earlier and not drink so much, thus being a bit more on the ball when it came to handling explosives and working with the antiquated machinery which Britain's factory entrepreneurs had not sufficiently upgraded.

What was popularly known as the Munitions Act established the Liquor Traffic Control Board and what followed was a heavy tax on drink. In 1915 (when, incidentally, it was still legal to buy cocaine and opium in Harrods!) the Board put a stop to the 19.5 hours opening time in London (17 hours in the provinces) and replaced it with just 5.5 hours opening times with a two hour closure from midday.

The Allies went on to win the war. Statistics show that these initiatives led to a dramatic decline in drunkenness. Such a drastic reduction in opening times was always going to lead to this but it also needs to be remembered that millions of potential drinkers were being shelled to death across the Channel thus greatly reducing their opportunity for any public drunkenness in the UK.

In 1918 and 1919, drunkenness increased but then drifted downwards, so much so that in 1921 the opening hours were extended to nine hours a day in London and eight elsewhere.

Gin drinking decreased between the wars, as did drunkenness arrests but interestingly beer consumption edged up year on year.

The Second World War came and went, significantly reducing populations around the world and leaving most countries in a perilous economic state. In Britain, life had changed forever. Rationing remained in place for many years but having trained and armed the general population, it was clear to the authorities and to the government that many things had to change.

A health service, housing, employment and education all had to be accessible for all. The resultant NHS was radically different to the one originally envisaged run by the medical establishment. This meant that health was treated as a medical intervention rather than rooted in social circumstances. It reinforced the notion of individual rather than holistic diagnosis. For alcohol misuse it reinforced the individual illness approach.

To this day, the individual is responsible for their drinking and subsequent problems, and the supply can only be controlled by central government through either supply or price.

In the 1950s, Britain was probably as sober as it had ever been. Now it was time for Alcoholic Anonymous to make its entrance to Britain. It was introduced to the UK in the late 1940s from America. The main protagonist was W.D. Silkworth, who proposed that alcoholism was an allergy to alcohol, with the drinking becoming the disease process. Thus once the disease was contracted it could not be cured, it could only be held in abeyance by not drinking.

It sounds like temperance in new clothes but, no, the Temperance Movement was still alive and kicking and still campaigning. The AA movement was very different. It was not a campaigning movement. It was not about setting an example to others. The main premise was the idea that fellow drinkers could talk to each other and to help each other to maintain sobriety. It was a self-help group, independent of professional help. Secondly, it was anonymous. In the absence of any decent treatment alternatives it was a wonderful idea to many people.

To the government and the drinks industry it must have felt like 'manna from heaven'. Here was a self-help group that did not cost public money and had an approach that 'preached' individual illness and responsibility. Neither was it political.

In the 1960s, the medical world and AA came together with E. Morton Jellinek's book *The Disease Concept of Alcoholism*. Much of the work was based on research from AA. In the book, the alcohol problem was neatly categorised and given medical terminology. It was oddly named after letters of the Greek alphabet and based on levels of dependency and severity:

Alpha alcoholism - this was psychological dependence on alcohol.
Beta alcoholism - there is no psychological or physical dependence but there is physical damage – development of cirrhosis, digestive problems and so forth.
Gamma alcoholism – there is an increased shift to physical dependence which if the drinking is interrupted will lead to withdrawal symptoms. There is a loss of control.
Delta alcoholism – his classification describes this as the same as Gamma but the drinker has control of what s/he consumes. However, any attempt at stopping leads to severe withdrawals.
Epsilon alcoholism – Jellinek describes this as periodic alcoholism. This has led to many describing it as binge drinking (Jellinek referred to it as periodic drinking).

This was his attempt to bring a type of science to what was previously based on belief.

It described alcoholism as a disease. Merged with the belief of what had gone before, we were then left with the notion that it is a disease that can never be cured but merely held in abeyance by not drinking. Individuals are never recovered but in a permanent state of recovering.

Today's new drug and alcohol strategy has to be considered in this context – periodic drinking is often described as bingeing, despite the official classification of bingeing beginning at over four units (around two pints of lager depending on strength), which I am sure is not what Jellinek was thinking at the time.

More concerning is that the whole treatment strategy is targeting people to recovery – abstinence from drugs and from alcohol and the treatment service does not receive payment for a part of their treatment unless this happens (more of which later)

It laid the foundation for treatment of alcoholism – that of individual self-induced illness. In 1962, the Ministry of Health set up the first alcohol treatment unit in Warlingham Park Hospital, Surrey, under Dr Max Glatt.

By 1977, there were thirty six of these units in the country. Harm reduction was to stop drinking alcohol completely. It was the only treatment and the self-help and mutual talking support of AA had become the talking therapy of groups and individual counselling of the medical world.

From here came a proliferation of organisations – the Medical Council on Alcoholism and the Alcohol Education Centre (based at the Maudsley Hospital) and the National Council on Alcoholism.

What caused a sensation in the early 1970s was the publication of Mark and Linda Sobells' paper on controlled drinking. This paper was met with almost heretical hysteria. The Sobells proposed that alcohol was not a disease whose only solution was to hold it abeyance through abstinence, but that individuals could be taught to reduce their consumption and the harm associated with it.

What spread from here was a proliferation of treatment options and reconsidering drinking as a continuum from social to heavy to problematic to dependent drinking; it split the notion between psychological dependence and physical dependence. The government got in on the act in the 1980s and 1990s with terms like 'sensible drinking', units of alcohol, price controls and so forth. By the 1980s, the Treasury income ran into the billions from the sale of alcohol through duty, tax and licensing. Members of Parliament were sponsored by the brewers; the industry was a huge employer. Drinks were increasingly advertised everywhere.

This was all happening in the complete vacuum of any strategic approach by government on drinking and alcohol.

Through the '80s and '90s drinking levels increased dramatically and by the late '90s and new years of the new century, the drinking levels, price, availability and drunkenness reached saturation point. A national alcohol strategy – Alcohol Harm Reduction Strategy for England and Wales arrived. Not only did it have an unfortunate acronym (if you drop Wales) – AHRSE but it arrived after the Licensing Act, which finally overhauled the Munitions Act of 1915 in terms of opening hours. There was no money to support the Strategy (unlike the National Drugs Strategy), no person to lead it and it has continued to muddy the waters of social, health and criminal justice policy on alcohol.

That's it – a brief history of alcohol misuse and the approaches to trying to tackle the biggest health, social and criminal justice problem that the UK faces.

"This sceptred isle, whose cup never overfloweth because there is always a drunk bingeing from it, has the reputation of drunkenness.

As Britain's standing in the world wanes from the Commonwealth and the Military, from Financial Centre and the Mother of Parliaments, it has replaced it as the increasing drunk of the world. Where it used to be limited to Football and Spain, with the aid of Easy Jet and Ryanair, we have exported tourism drunkenness to every capital in Europe and beyond."

— A good friend having a wonderful rant

CHAPTER THREE

TERMINOLOGY AND TREATMENT

So far we have covered the terminology our public health and government officials like us to use. These are 'sensible drinking levels', 'drinking responsibly', 'bingeing', and 'at risk drinking', 'heavy drinking' and 'dependent drinker'.

Now let's throw a few more in that are a mix of the new and the old:

Alcoholic, Lush, Drunk, Drunkard, Recovering Alcoholic, Social Drinker, Heavy Drinker, Street Drinker, Barfly, Dipsomania, Vagrant, Psychologically Addicted, Physically Addicted.

And how do we describe our drinking?

Drunk, Rotten, Stocious, Full, Pissed, Blathered, Rat-arsed

And how do we describe what happens?

Blacked Out, Threw up (or Chucked up, Sick, Puked)

So how we describe our own behaviour and our friends is more than a little different to how our esteemed professionals describe our behaviour and the effects of drinking.

As I have previously stated, I do not know about you but when I go to the pub I do not want to be sensible or responsible.

Most of us have spent the day being responsible at work, with the family, driving and so forth and want to laugh, relax, talk and gossip. We want to be safe but certainly not sensible and responsible.

So why do they use sensible and responsible? To make sure that no one wants to read the message?

Why is the information that we are given, so different to our experience?

Having confused us with the messages of how to drink safely (units) and then with the terminology, which is utterly different to our everyday language, what happens when we then attach labels such as Heavy Drinker, Dependent Drinker, Alcoholic?

Not surprisingly, behind all this confusion and the muddled history of what to do over the centuries, we have another mini industry of treatment, all of whom will argue that their approach is the most valid.

There is a section in this book that describes these treatment options. Suffice to say, however, the diagnosis and who is it is absolutely crucial to what then happens to that individual.

The three choices anyone has is either to cut down on their drinking, to cease drinking (and become abstinent), or to change or cease the behaviour and drinking that is problematic or a danger, by, for example, walking or getting a taxi to the pub rather than driving.

What the professional does with their diagnostic label is to determine which of those options is available to the person drinking. Once the label is attached, then there is a set of rules and expectations that comes with the diagnosis.

All of this happens despite what the individual may think. The effect is that they will be further labelled as either being in denial or resistant to change or treatment.

Straying from those expectations and rules brings a further set of labels and descriptions – the professionals call it a relapse;

Self Help Groups will describe it as a slip or—worse—that the person has not yet reached rock bottom. The person at the centre of all this feels a failure, whilst struggling with this label and new set of rules.

Now of course there are many individuals who knew their drinking was problematic to them or out of control and treatment and help has arrived at exactly the right time. However for many, they have been labelled with a chronic disorder, they have been told how to behave (the new 24/7 sobriety programme as a sentencing option instead of prison is an example of this) and how to think and how to behave differently, all without a drug that they have relied on and have been a huge part of their life. Expecting even 10 per cent of these people to succeed straight away is like expecting some kind of biblical miracle.

CHAPTER FOUR

HARM REDUCTION AND THE PUB
(LICENSED PREMISES AND THE TRADE IN GENERAL)

Probably the best health message on any alcoholic beverage appears on Cyprus's beer Keo: BE HAPPY AND DRINK WELL. It surely conveys what having a drink is all about.

Having had a long career of trying to promote harm reduction, my experiences are usually reduced to running stalls at markets and health awareness events, usually with colleagues in T-shirts that were either far too big or way too small; usually with a poor design but with the result that we either looked like the Michelin Man (when they are too small) or someone who has a heinous disease involving rapid weight loss.

Harm Reduction advice has to start at source, in the licensed premises across the UK.

However, when we talk about the drinks industry – what do we mean? There are the producers of alcoholic beverages, the companies who make the beer, lager, wine, spirits, cider, liquors and so forth. Then there are those who run the licensed premises in terms of public houses and clubs, there is everyone who has a licence to sell alcohol, which is now not just the big supermarket chains but virtually every corner shop.

It is a big supply chain with a complicated financial structure and regulatory system, with a huge socio-economic influence.

These various components of the 'industry' range from multi-national companies who have diversified across many products and markets in addition to alcoholic products and have a range of representative bodies now makes a big thing of how they promote sensible or responsible drinking. This book has already covered the issue that it is perhaps the Treasury that presents the biggest barrier to change and this chapter sets out how harm reduction can be practised coherently by the trade/ industry, and dares to suggest that maybe if it had a more balanced role with Public Health and the fighting stopped then perhaps, just perhaps, we might all be in a better place.

Drinking should be an enjoyable experience. If it is not an enjoyable experience for the drinker or those who live with them then there is a problem. It really is that simple.

It is so simple that we forget this.

We remain ambivalent about our drinking. We neither act positively about tackling the harms nor are we positive about drinking as a nation. There is almost a denial, especially amongst health and social policy, from practitioners about being positive about it.

Instead, huge swathes of people drink to excess and behave in ways that we choose not to when not drinking. This then encourages the stereotype of our drinking culture and those who lean to control, regulate and to moralise come to the fore.

As we will discussed earlier, this confusion is stark when it comes to how to induct young people into the culture of the UK around drinking practices and beliefs.

Finally, as also previously covered, the issue with units of alcohol highlights the obsession we have with levels of consumption, rather than behaviour and drinking. The incidence of disorder and violence (physical and verbal) and drinking is not linked to a linear progression of drinking. There may be for accidents but not disorder.

The overall alcohol industry, including the pubs, is not interested in reducing consumption neither for economic reasons, nor from a harm reduction point of view. Their very strong interest is reducing the harm of violence, anti-social behaviour and theft on their properties.

Let me give you a quote by Colin Dexter (1992):

The pub is a separate circle of existence. You have your job, your family, circles that intertwine and overlap, but the pub is somehow outside that. It's another little world – like going to another country but not very far away. It's a different ambience, a sense of independence, and that sort of feeling is very valuable. Above all, for me, it is the magic combination of friendship, conversation and beer – that form together a sort of alchemy of a very enjoyable piece of existence.

Over the last 10 to 15 years, this ideal has changed for many within the towns and cities, as regeneration has created larger and larger drinking establishments (it is hard to call them pubs) with an emphasis on vertical drinking rather than being seated. As we noted in the section on Regeneration, we have seen some of our churches, chapels, banks and even libraries and cinemas converted into large bars and often clustered together along the same part of town.

At the same time, the traditional image of the Public House has started to disappear. Many rural and town pubs have had to close as they have become uneconomic. The majority who have survived have rebranded themselves as public house and restaurant, or have become a Carvery.

The concept of binge drinking has also become an issue over the last 10 to 15 years and is again something that has caused massive confusion and debate.

On the one hand, we have had a growing pre-occupation with drinking as much as possible and as fast as we can, whilst on the other hand the government suggests that a binge is drinking over four units of alcohol in one session (which is two pints of lager). The targets for blame have been with parts of the drinks industry with Happy Hour and other discount promotions.

This, the retail trade argue, is to encourage people to come in and drink earlier rather than staying at home and drinking (and getting drunk) on much cheaper drink that is available from the supermarkets and local shops. Either way, the outcome in the city centre is usually drunken mayhem.

The cycle of 'tough talking' by the politicians and the various measures introduced has the effect of backing the licensees, the drink companies, the police and the local authorities all into their own corners and blaming one another. Throw our health watch dogs into the mix who say ban happy hours and stop the supermarkets selling cheap alcohol. The politicians will point out that the laws are already there for the police and local authority to enforce and the supermarkets will quite rightly argue that what they price any product is up to them.

For me, as I have said previously, it is reminiscent of the deck chairs being re-arranged on the deck of the Titanic.

So what to say about the supermarkets and retail outlets that represent a major part of our drinks industry?

Bargain Booze shopping chain – the name says it all. They are purveyors of cheap alcohol. Love them or loathe them, they are legally selling alcoholic beverages. As we have said, supermarkets sell cheap alcohol, sometimes at promotional prices below cost but they also sell a range of quality alcoholic beverages.

If the traditional corner shop is to survive anywhere, especially on estates, then they need to sell cheap drinks to attract customers in order to survive. Therefore, all corner shops need to have a licence to sell alcohol.

Who decides who can have a licence and who cannot?
Magistrates.
Who can object?
Anyone.

On what grounds can they object?
Whether the licensee is fit and proper.

So there laid out before us is the issue – no one can object on any other grounds apart from being near a school or other such technical issues. A local authority has no grounds to say that it has enough licensed premises in any one locality or borough.

But also let us get back to the good and the bad of the public houses. They can be the hub of preparing anti-social disorder. Some public houses have a history of being places of disrepute. Let's face it, some licensed premises are badly run, consistently break the law and should be closed down by the local authorities and police (who already have the powers to do so but choose on the whole not to).

On the other hand, both in towns and in rural places, pubs are seen as a hub of the community, they are places for people to mix and interact; some pubs are where tradesmen meet and do business. Historically it is where freemasons and friendly societies were formed, with rooms where social reformers, clubs, weddings and meetings take place, where live music can be listened to.

So what to do about Harm Reduction in the pub?

- Information on drinking advice should be freely available.
- An Information Board giving advice and help should be compulsory.
- Stronger enforcement of not selling to those heavily intoxicated could be more strongly promoted.
- Decent non-alcoholic beverages need to be more widely available and at a price that is favourable to beer prices.
- Making pubs more integrated with their communities, especially rurally (post offices, meetings for clubs, etc.).
- Make lower strength beer and lager cheaper in comparison.
- Link up with local health services – GPs, nurses.

- Strong local initiatives around anti-social behaviour. Build on Pub Watch, give the licensees a stronger local responsibility with the local authority.
- Allow health services to have access to advertising space for a range of alcohol-related disorders.
- Review the licensed premises that have an excess of standing area to seated area.
- Recognise the very lack of real alternatives to the pub as a hub and make them more open. For young people – what has happened to all out playing fields, how expensive have swimming pools and fitness clubs become? Access to music and creative venues of the arts and developing talent – where are the alternatives? Where are the alternatives to drinking?

These are all small steps but behind them is the call for a radical rethink and overhaul on how local partnerships work and what can be done to foster a step change in how we deal with anti-social behaviour, as a result of drinking.

It needs to be linked with a change in how we view drinking and the style in which we drink. Going to the pub should be fun and a good experience, whether we are drinking alcohol or not. We all want to be safe but not sensible in the pub and there is a part of every adult that can relate to Colin Dexter's quote, obviously with a bit more 'uummphhh' if you are younger.

In writing this chapter I would like to express my appreciation of three gentlemen who have had the honesty and courage to talk about many of these issues, who have all enjoyed long careers working in the treatment of problematic drinking and who greatly influenced me – Ron McKechie, Doug Cameron and Trevor McCarthy from the New Directions in the Study of Alcohol (and as CAMRA Members).

In closing I also want to say that Ron McKechie sadly left this world while I was writing this book and I never managed to ask him to read it – I hope Ron you have found your perfect pub with good company and banter and good beer and a wee dram of malt for the journey home each night.

CHAPTER FIVE

WHAT DO WE MEAN BY HARM REDUCTION OR REDUCING THE HARM?

Harm Reduction is simple. We are talking about anything that reduces the harm associated with drinking and drinking too much.

Harm Reduction is about cutting down overall consumption of alcohol, either over a week or on a daily basis, or eventually stopping altogether for a period of time or forever.

Harm Reduction is about being able to self-risk assess and to avoid certain behaviours or actions when drinking.

Harm Reduction is about improving physical and mental health. It is about drinking less but learning to eat more healthily, take exercise and to replace drinking habits with other activities that make you feel better about yourself.

Harm Reduction is about addressing issues that might be worrying you – relationships, debts, legal issues, work issues, health concerns and injuries.

Harm Reduction is about self-development and learning.

Harm Reduction is about taking on responsibilities for oneself or others.

Harm Reduction is about reducing the amount of the drug called alcohol that you drink AND about EVERYTHING ELSE. It is not Rocket Science.

Harm Reduction is about both achieving abstinence and cutting down on consumption

Cutting down or cutting out drinking alcohol may be an achievement in itself but if it leaves you feeling miserable or depressed, being obsessed about not drinking, short tempered, feeling bored or edgy or anxious, then you are unlikely to sustain the gains you have made.

Harm Reduction is therefore importantly about making lifestyle changes.

A Natural Change Process

There should be a growing acceptance that for someone with severe alcohol misuse can take over seven years to completely change or turn their lives around after accepting that they have a problem which needs addressing. That is what the evidence tells me from watching people overcome their problems over the last 30 years.

The problem is whether the treatment and commissioning system is doing something wrong? There are many people who have become disaffected with a system that is not providing the right support and services for them. It then becomes easy to place the entire responsibility onto the individual and if s/he falls short of the system's expectations then the blame falls on them as well.

In working in a harm reduction manner, a significant amount of alcohol treatment works within the Cognitive Behavioural Treatment approach, which considers basically 'how the brain works' with its thinking and how it responds to the environment and experience and behaves accordingly.

Part of the CBT approach is the cycle of change (again featured later in more detail), which considers that the brain receives feedback, considers the issues and decides whether to go and action some change or revert to previous behaviour.

To do this with a learnt behaviour and all the arguments going on in the head (it's called dissonance for the intellectuals) then some very serious arguments have to happen internally and the brain needs to find plenty of excuses not to change. When the argument is lost, then the dysfunctional thinking has to look for excuses to revert back to old behaviour and looks for what we call triggers to take you off drinking again – domestic arguments, stress at work, no work, the train was late, the cat pissed behind the TV, 'I feel depressed' and so forth.

That gives the platform to go drinking and then, after the initial brief honeymoon of drink, the guilt and remorse kicks in and the arguments start up again the head.

So it is no surprise then that this 'debate' takes ages to start to be resolved. Even harder still is persuading oneself to then action some change because it involves facing up to bad feelings, talking about it, carrying out tasks you would rather not do and if that was not enough, cutting down or abandoning your security blanket – drinking alcohol. For those physically addicted, there is also the bodily reaction of withdrawing, which is usually worse than any illicit drug or medication in the short term.

Little wonder that for many, this is a Herculean task, especially as for most of us life is never plain sailing at the best of times. As Mao said, a long journey starts with the first step but he never talked about going naked (emotionally) as well.

Anyhow, parallel to all this is the positive side – the person begins to get sick of drinking, bored of the same routine and sick and tired of the arguments in the head. For some this is it, time for a change, for others it becomes a time of reflection and possible action and of course for others the behaviour is just repeated and like many things, an awful lot of thinking and words but no action.

This is where the next key 'treatment' thing kicks in. Motivational Interviewing (MI) is what a lot of us do on occasion with friends and family until the need to take control and be directive or blaming or opinionated takes over. MI is designed to enable professionals to assist the person in reflecting on what they are saying and to pull out key aspects and let the person build on it, look at solutions, consider thoughts from a constructive standpoint, consider what could be done but all through their own volition. When you see it done by someone who is skilled at it, it is very impressive.

But back to where this part started and a natural recovery can take and usually does take years. After all of the above then there is the guilt to start to come to terms with, the broken promises and let downs, staying away from drinking companions, avoiding triggers.

In terms of harm reduction to the general population what the British Medical Association (BMA) argue, is that there is a need to cut overall consumption. The tools for doing this are to raise prices (they advocate a standard minimum price per unit of alcohol - this makes stronger drinks, like strong lagers, more expensive). This would then be backed up by stronger control of the licensed premises in terms of promotions and running of the establishments, with enforced closure or suspensions of licence if the establishment becomes problematic.

In later chapters you will read why I clearly do not concur with this approach. As stated elsewhere, the BMA also view the general population as largely homogenous. It is difficult to obtain a clear consensus on the research on drinking over sensible levels and its impact on future health. Some studies indicate an increase in hypertension, accidents and financial concerns but acknowledge that this could be linked to other pressures and dynamics. There is a strong link between constant excessive drinking and liver cirrhosis but a number of studies which look at alcohol consumption over recommended safe limits are not conclusive at all and, as I indicate in later chapters, this is more likely to be linked to individual health, social, genetic and environmental factors.

The bottom line is that if you drink too much all the time, then of course you are going to have health difficulties, of course your loved ones are going to get pissed off, could lead to financial pressures and yes, being pissed will make you more accident prone and at risk from others. It's not rocket science – it's the bleeding obvious and it seems to me that everyone has forgotten that.

A little word about recovery and recovering

Recovery is a word that has appeared in the lexicon of drinking and alcohol use/abuse. In fact it has become the new foundation stone of the whole treatment movement, after the National Treatment Agency switched from retention in treatment as the goal to recovery being the goal (after significant pressure and criticism from various 'think tanks' and lobbying groups that drug users were stuck in treatment and that retention was no longer a good thing).

Recovery is now enshrined in the new government Drug and Alcohol Treatment Strategy.

Recovery for me is something like recovering from a cold or a car has been recovered from where it broke down. It is also a word that is strongly associated with the whole Alcoholics Anonymous approach, with all the implications that comes with this. The essential difference is that in AA, people will refer to themselves as in recovery or as recovering alcoholics.

Recovery within drinking has its basis historically in the notion that a person has reached their 'rock bottom' (their worst moment) and is slowly ascending from the bottom of the pit in which they descended and is on the steep and difficult path of recovering.

It is akin to salvation and has much to liken it to religious conversion. It is about the reclaiming of one's soul and about improving one's life. For many it is easy to explain in relation to spiritual change and does not necessarily have to carry a religious connotation.

In working with people who drink, many of us have tried hard to support people who are making changes to their lives, as simple processes, a change in behaviour or belief. Not to create labels or banner headlines, not to set themselves up with grand changes. This long journey starts with the classic first step and this is what harm reduction is all about because once the first step is taken then there is a world of possibilities, not just one road to recovery and salvation.

I have included this little section because much of the treatment of alcohol and drugs has not so much been hijacked by the term 'recovery' but hijacked itself. Once the National Treatment Agency confirmed its preference for the term 'recovery' in its next forward strategic approach, then the treatment agencies, like any modern company in any market, ignoring their carefully constructed charitable terminology simply inserted the term 'recovery' somewhere in a strap line or their ethos description. As a result nearly all the major 'charities' have jumped on the bandwagon of Recovery - that this is the only way - to stop and recover from their addiction and disease. The new government appears to want to back this with payment for treatment by results. This brave new world may work for a minority but for the majority changing their drinking and behaviour may take a very long time and may not be easy. Not achieving abstinence in such a national model and construct of recovery makes the sense of failure more acute.

What is this place called 'Recovery'? Do they not mean 'Recovered'? At least recovered implies that the problem is resolved once and for all. Recovered is what the strategy is really referring to and it is what is implied in 'Payment by Results'. Treatment services do not receive their full funding, unless the client has signed up to the pledge of abstinence and achieved it for at least six months.

The term Recovery began to appear in the drug treatment field because of funding issues. Residential Rehabilitation schemes and 12 step Treatment Services (modelled on the steps in AA) were finding themselves increasingly starved of funding because the commissioning bodies saw them as increasingly expensive compared to community based treatment options and even more expensive compared with prescribing services, where clients could be held in services with sufficient numbers that demonstrated so called cost efficient services (please note that this is not cost effective services). The so called Models of Care, alongside the entire treatment field moving to competitive tendering, meant that unless the politics changed, then many of these residential rehabilitation and 12 step services were going to go out of business.

Part of the back lash was the suggestion that too many people were trapped within the prescribing treatment services. In the UK there exists among some commentators, the idea that much of the harm reduction work was at worst encouraging continued drug use and certainly not addressing any reduction in drug use.

With the previous Labour government having invested much time and money into the Drugs Strategy, and with the likelihood of losing office in the next General Election, the Drugs Strategy started to change and Recovery started to enter the lexicon. Like a hole in the dam, a trickle turned into a deluge and the entire drug treatment strategy changed course.

Come the General Election and enter a coalition under Prime Minister Cameron and political and economic expediency took over. The new drug treatment strategy included alcohol. Alcohol treatment now had Recovery at centre stage as well as drugs.

Payment by Results

I was particularly struck by Payment by Results. It was proposed and is now being tested in six areas and will roll out across the country because the strategy says it will (even though it is theoretically still being tested for effectiveness).

The question is this - when did the treatment field decide that it was them who stopped people taking drugs and alcohol?

From everything I have ever experienced, from every person who has had a drink problem no matter how mild or severe, from autobiographies of drinkers and any research findings I have read, I always thought that ultimately it was the individual who decided for themselves whether to stop or carry on.

The treatment field was often there supporting and assisting them in this process, helping to manage a crisis with a detoxification or a hostel. Advocating on their behalf; making referrals to GPs; sometimes, just showing you had a belief in them when no one else did.

In some programmes we are able to give individuals tools to understand their cognitive processes better or insight into their behaviour or destructive relationships. We can teach individuals to understand what risky situations are and how to avoid them. It is all valuable 'stuff' to arm someone with to help combat their problems. These examples though are not 'stopping' someone drinking, nor are they ensuring so called 'recovery'

I was not aware that anyone possessed the ability to stop someone drinking. I guess if there was such ability, then there might be a mention in the Bible or somewhere similar (because it would certainly be on a par with turning water into wine or numerous other 'miracles'). In my experience not even counsellors laid claim to such abilities.

Generally though, I never worked with anyone who felt that superior or blessed enough to be able to do this. Clearly there are now a number of Chief Executives of treatment agencies and some of their staff (along with Commissioners and those in government) who do believe they have these 'super powers' (as I would describe them).

So, not content with abandoning their charitable aims and objectives they are now playing God to clients and appear to have rejected any coherence that addiction to alcohol and drugs can be a chronic relapsing disorder, which renders the whole recovery agenda a farce (especially as AA and NA strongly hold onto the fact that you are never recovered but recovering) - so presumably the penalty for anyone caught going to AA is to have a commissioner stopping the cheque payable to Recovery Incorporated (or whatever the treatment agency now calls itself) because by default they are still recovering rather than in recovery.

To some readers, this may sound pedantic, but a theme throughout this tome and throughout the issue of drinking is terminology and labelling, and this is one more step but this time a step too far. It is a step that has frightening consequences for individuals with drink and drug problems, civil liberties and the right to not only treatment but appropriate treatment.

For me, it represents the truth that treatment services view income generation through agreed contractual treatment outcome as more important than client need and what their achievable goals and outcomes can be.

To understand the social construct of being someone with an addiction and how you can end up being treated within the construct of Recovery, these notes I took from a presentation by John B Davies at a New Directions in the Study of Alcohol Group Conference are terribly relevant.

John B Davies is a Professor at the University of Glasgow, who has inspired many of us who work with alcohol use and misuse. These notes do not reflect the dexterity of his thinking but are an important note to anyone trying to help or work with someone whose drinking is problematic.

In a nutshell, we may be presented with an array of individuals with their own individual stories about their drinking but essentially these stories boil down to some very simple concepts:

Reflexes are not actions. They are evoked responses.
Reflexes have physiological/pharmacological causes.
There is 'no story' to a knee jerk. A knee jerk has a cause but no reason.
Drinking is an action. You do it. It does not happen to you.
Therefore every drinking habit has a reason.
Reasons build into a story / stories.
Everyone has their own individual story (a personal story built around pleasure/pain). This personal story is built around a core which everyone has.
The fusion of individual habits and core stories produce a narrative.
These narratives are good and bad stories.

Good stories tend to have a few, strong explanations.
Bad stories tend to have lots of weak explanations.
Explaining success have few explanations.
Explaining failure have lots of excuses/reasons.

The 'Core Story' – the story of alcoholism is in general circulation. It is a biography of symptoms. It is socially constructed and everyone knows it. It a story, not an act or personal recall. People who cannot remember their drinking from yesterday can tell a perfect story. They choose when, where and whether to "tell their tale".

From his observations of men and women in treatment he notes that:

There appears to be two scripts – one for a Social drinker and one for a Problem Drinker. They fill in two questionnaires, each one describing what it is like to be a SD or PD.

Drinkers who stay in treatment have a different index of sensitivity towards normal drinking than those who drop out. The ones that drop out did not show that sensitivity.

To add to John's observations, we need to understand that Treatment is within a social construct, rather than in terms of individual need.

The drinker is guilty, sinful, easy to punish, weak, able to be rejected. The public/society cannot respond rationally and as a consequence a great deal of interventions cannot respond rationally.

Public opinion is embedded within the culture and as a result the responses represent this. As a consequence, drinkers (along with drug users) are as a group blamed and punished, through our criminal justice processes. Around 70 per cent of the prison population have a mix of alcohol, drugs and mental health problems.

Even if this group elicit some aspect of sympathy or understanding, ultimately our cultural beliefs result in negative responses. This group then offers itself as a scapegoat for much of our society ills (certainly in excess to the reality).

PART TWO

IT'S NOT ROCKET SCIENCE

Introduction

The second section of this book is for everyone—people who drink who want to cut down, or learn and understand more, people who work with those who drink, family and friends of drinkers, people in professions across the board. Somewhere in this section there is something for everyone. It will try to assist on how to drink with less dangerous consequences; how to enjoy the benefits over the harms; how to cut down and even stop (temporarily or for the long term); how to replace drinking behaviour, and finally how to watch out for tripping yourself up (relapse prevention) and returning to old behaviour.

If your drinking, or the drinking of someone close to you, has reached a point where the harms outweigh the benefits, or if you are worried about your drinking or simply want to cut down, then these chapters are hopefully designed for you.

Similarly, if you are a relative, partner or friend then again, hopefully these pages will offer insight and practical tips on helping someone else.

Lastly, if you are in contact with someone who is drinking because you are a professional working with them, I hope these pages may help you recognise that their drinking may need to be addressed and is more importantly intimately related to the problem that you are dealing with or trying to manage.

Furthermore, whatever strategy or tool you have to hand may be ineffective until the drinking is addressed.

What is important is that between us all we try to help and arrest the problematic drinking.

Because what is important to understand from the first part of this book, no one else is going to – certainly not our elected officials and certainly not the Ministries that operate under them. They will all talk tough and tell us how concerned they are but in reality they will do nothing, mainly because they do not know how to, but also because they are only in office for a maximum of 5 years and trying to tackle and untangle the mess we are in within the silo of thinking and government strategies of alcohol, drugs and tobacco cannot happen overnight.

CHAPTER SIX

IT'S NOT ROCKET SCIENCE – BASIC ADVICE

What is alcohol?

Alcohol is a legal drug. It is a depressant drug. As a depressant drug it dampens down the central nervous system. In other words it slows down how you work. This fundamental effect is difficult to understand at first because of the contradictory effects.

What does it do to you?

After a couple of drinks you will begin to feel more relaxed and less anxious. Whether alone or in company, the world will feel a slightly better place and your optimism for it will be better. Your mood will lift. This is the drug suppressing your central nervous system, making you more relaxed, less anxious. After some more alcohol then the drug will begin to effectively suppress the parts of the brain that control things like judgement and physical coordination.

In terms of judgement, a little bit of self-delusion comes in – you feel not only better but perhaps a little thinner (if you think you weigh too much), perhaps not as bald or spotty, your bum does not look so big in those trousers. Suddenly, the bar staff are looking prettier or handsome and perhaps that vacant look from someone at the next table is a meaningful look (of course after many more drinks that vacant look may well be interpreted as 'what are you looking at?').

The inhibitions begin to go – boring stories and conversation become more interesting or funnier. How many times do you hear friends laughing about something that is not that funny at all, when drink has been taken? Sometimes you become louder, more physical in your articulation – you flirt more.

Then the physical coordination becomes a little affected – it is why it is never a good idea to drink and drive. Over 50 milligrams it is of course illegal but before that your judgement will be slightly impaired; your reaction times will be slower; your concentration not so good. Just half a second slower at around 40 mph and it is the difference between braking in time to miss the pedestrian who has stepped off the kerb without looking and hitting them, because it equates to about 30 metres.

Your balance may be a little off after the third, fourth or fifth drink; your words do not come out so easily, your vision can be a little blurred. You can become clumsy. It is round about this time that drinks get knocked over or spilled, you stop paying attention to the handbag or lap top under the table and when you come back from the loo – it's gone!

Depending on the circumstances, after the sixth, seventh or eighth drink and beyond, it's a route to anything from hiccups and nausea, to raised voices and arguing, from swaying and falling over, memory loss and anger to vomiting, passing out, becoming abusive or just falling asleep.

Some people will be able to carry on drinking – it depends on the individual. A bottle of wine is around 4 to 5 glasses (though a pub measure glass will either be a standard for around 6 glasses or a large which will account for a bottle in around 3/3.5 glasses). A bottle of vodka has about 32 shots in it or around 16 doubles.

There is no consistency in plotting this process. Some will just carry on laughing or being funny. They will be the life and soul of the party, want to carry on drinking. It really is a very personal relationship with drink. We can predict and chart likelihood of behaviour, likely effect on the brain and body but it is not a blanket thing. Nor is it a competition about who can hold their drink better. How some people behave when drinking, the best advice is not to drink at all.

What is fundamentally important is that we all learn to understand our own personal relationship between ourselves and alcohol and the types of alcoholic beverages we drink. It is not until anyone reaches that point that you can then be honest about that relationship if you are to avoid the harm. However, like any relationship, there is always the capacity to be surprised or affected one day much more than you usually are.

The point is that you cannot just look at the volume going into the body and expect exactly the same reaction day in and day out. Inside our bodies are systems, organs and a brain that is constantly going through cycles, interacting with the environment and people, absorbing food, missing out on sleep.

Trying to get the balance right with all this, so you get the positives and not the negatives is the key to ensuring that harm does not come to you. This has to be learnt. How you learn this is through experience and education, through peers and family. How you are influenced to drink by advertising and how you are regulated to not drink all comes into the mix and finally, as has already been stated, how you react personally to the taste and effect of different alcoholic drinks all come into play.

I have heard older men (from Scotland and Ireland) at weddings and family functions talk about not drinking spirits because in their younger years - 'the fists have come up with drink'. However, come a wake, then the drinking of spirits would be expected.

Women will often say that drinking a bottle of wine in a pub will 'get them pissed' while drinking the same amount at home they would be OK.

Drinking strong lagers often seems to encourage raucous and rowdy behaviour. Wine drinkers and Real Ale imbibers do not appear to come out fighting. Are these ridiculous examples of stereotyping, or do they have a basis of truth? Does a certain drink product suit a certain personality? Do some drinks encourage us to drink in certain ways because we have learnt this through our culture? Do we choose a type of drink to suit our moods or to behave in a certain way? I have often heard violence being excused because the perpetrator had been drinking spirits.

Of course, as has already been hinted at, overlapping all of this are the cultural, political and moral attitudes that influence and mould our drinking behaviour and attitudes.

Clearly the very simple message of only having about 5 or 6 pints of lager or a bottle and a half of wine a week as a man and even less as a woman and to spread it out over seven days and to have two to four days without alcohol and not drive, is very sensible and it is likely that little or no harm will come to you in relation to drink related harm.

The reality of this makes for a very guarded and watchful lifestyle, and how many of us go out for an evening and have only one or two drinks? Moreover, it is not that simple – someone can have an alcohol-related accident after two drinks and alcohol-related domestic violence is not limited to the quantity of alcohol drunk – it is a much more complicated interaction.

Returning to the contradictions of the good and bad effects - a few drinks can lead to intimacy and even sex, it can make the least confident person confident and the dullest person feel funny, the unwanted person wanted, the lonely it can give company.

One to many and all those negative feelings can be multiplied ten times or allow things to spiral out of control –

unsafe sex or forced sex, fighting and arguing, embarrassment, becoming ill, physical harm, accident (yes you are seven times more likely to have an accident), theft, you lose your belongings – the list is various and almost endless.

Accidental endgame

It can even lead to death – accidents, choking on your vomit, a victim of stranger violence, walking in front of traffic, falling off the platform, thinking you are Mr or Mrs Invincible – most drowning incidents are alcohol-related. Something like 86 per cent of murders involve drinking alcohol (and 80 per cent of murders are committed by a person known to the victim – so drinking with a relative is statistically a high risk leisure activity).

You will find plenty of information about all this in adverts, manuals, reports and educational material which you can usually pick up in doctor's surgeries and clinics, in council offices and so forth but never in the pub or bar. You may not read them while you are drinking, when your judgement is coming under the influence. This is why you need to be armed with some tactics which you feel comfortable with.

They also unfortunately start with the words 'sensible' or 'responsibly'. In all honesty, they might as well use the term 'boring' or at best just not use any description – just the facts and let us make up our minds.

These might sound simple but they work:

Take £10 out instead of £20.

Don't drink in Rounds.

Go out at 9.00 instead of 8.00 pm.

Drink less strong lager.

Drink wine with soda water or lemonade.

Alternate a wine or spirit with a soft drink and then back to the wine or spirit.

Stay off the spirits.

If you're thirsty, drink some water first, so you don't rush the first pint.

Set targets – not to have a drink before a certain time or event.

Try to avoid routines and learnt behaviour (a regular drink on the way home.

Have a few nights not drinking.

Don't drink if you are feeling angry, do something physical instead (no - not kicking the cat).

Do not drink immediately you are feeling stressed – learn some other tactics for that, like exercise, cooking, relaxation techniques, sex and if you want to drink a little later when you are calmer then you can.

CHAPTER SEVEN

IT'S NOT ROCKET SCIENCE – ADVICE FOR MORE SERIOUS CONCERNS

What do we mean when we talk about more serious concerns?

This book is about how to reduce the harm. It is about how to assess risk and to teach self-assessment of harmful risk and how to support those nearest and dearest.

A serious concern is when drinking affects health (physical and mental), family and personal relationships, housing, legal issues and offending, employment and unemployment issues, and debts. These problems are accumulative and not one off incidents or accidents.

Drinking excessively will impact on every aspect of life. Untangling the chicken and the egg or the other way around is a key for the longer term – did the drinking just increase or did other factors influence the drinking? What are the emotional triggers?

However, the reality of the situation is that if the drinking is heavy or serious then the associated problems are inextricably linked. It is not necessarily the amount but the style of drinking and how it impacts on their life.

Someone drinking daily a few beers or bottle of wine may encounter longer term health complications, then again they may not – it depends on general health, medication, diet, susceptibility to certain illnesses, the general state and functioning of the major organs of the body.

If they are in a relationship and the partner does not like it, or they drink to not communicate, for example, then you have drinking and relationship problems to untangle.

An excessive weekend of drinking could cause a Monday 'sickie', as it will have an impact on the body's organs (from irregular heartbeats, to damage to the lining of the stomach, to liver damage and, of course, alcohol speeds up the rate you lose brain cells), or it can lead to an accident, with concentration harder, clumsiness. If the weekend's drinking did not include the partner, wife or husband then it is unlikely to go down well at home.

For others going out on the 'tear' it can end in the police cell or A & E for an array of perpetrator or victim behaviours.

Domestic Violence

Domestic Violence is the same sorry tale – the perpetrator can have a couple of drinks or a bucketful – there is no level when it happens or stops. He or she may become angry because they are drinking and lose their inhibitions and turn to violence as an argument gets out of hand; for others they need the excuse of a drink in order to be violent.

The victim might drink and be unreasonable and intimidate or push and push an argument and a 'slap' happens to shut them up. For others this does not remain an occasional or 'one off' and becomes a learnt behaviour for both.

SIMPLE TIPS FOR CUTTING DOWN WITH SERIOUS CONCERNS

Switch from strong lager to a lesser strength lager.

Switch from spirits to beer or wine.

Start a drink diary – writing down when you drink and then look at patterns.

Be honest with yourself about your triggers for drinking.

Change your routines.

Start drinking ten minutes later each day (that is an hour over a week).

Try an alcohol free day (or two).

Start to fill each day with none drinking activities – walking, exercise, visits, clean the house, go shopping, and visit a friend.

Start taking more time on personal hygiene, your appearance and your clothes.

CHAPTER EIGHT

IT'S NOT ROCKET SCIENCE – ADVICE FOR WORKING WITH PEOPLE WITH OTHER SIGNIFICANT PROBLEMS

Drugs

Alcohol consumption among clients of drug services is well above the national average. This drinking is part of and in addition to the drug use. Therefore, attempting to discuss recommended safe drinking levels with clients is a relatively redundant process.

Unfortunately, for the last 15 years, most drug treatment services have ignored their clients' drinking. The only guidance in the early years of the National Treatment Agency within the National Drug Strategy was to actually produce information on sensible drinking for drug users. This for me was actually quite unbelievable advice to someone who is addicted to their drug use. Never mind that they were suggesting sensible drinking guidelines but that the assumption was that it was OK to drink at these levels when already using high levels of drugs and in many cases medication through scripts!

This document has been designed to consider drug using clients' drinking in relation to teaching and supporting risk behaviour and staff assessment. It will consider quantity in terms of daily intake but it will also consider what happens when drinking alcohol with drug use.

The National Treatment Outcome Research Study (NTORS) found that 33 per cent of those entering residential treatment or community methadone programmes were drinking at levels above those recommended as safe. Anecdotal evidence suggests that in London up to 50 per cent of clients on methadone prescriptions are 'physically addicted to alcohol'. It is likely that 75 to 80 per cent of clients of drug services are drinking above recommended safe levels. There is no way to prove this because the researched evidence is not available.

To compound this, drug workers are no different to many other professions who have an ambiguous attitude to alcohol and drinking themselves. Indeed, the Alcohol Harm Reduction Strategy for England (AHRSE) suggests that over 8 million of us drink over recommended safe levels.

The role of alcohol in offending behaviour and in terms of influencing cognition and poor risk behaviour, make it essential that **all** drug workers are competent and confident to talk about alcohol and drinking with their clients.

It is also a legal drug. It is a drug most individuals have taken to excess at some time. Most of us have a story where alcohol has played a part in shameful behaviour. However, most of us have far more stories where alcohol has played a part in good experiences. It is what makes us all so ambiguous about drinking and especially when someone is experiencing a problem with their drinking.

People who drink in addition to taking drugs are substantially more at risk. This is the same for prescription drugs and illegal drugs.

Heroin overdoses are far more likely to happen when the person is using and drinking.

Drink alcohol with cocaine (which is common) and the liver will break both down and produce a new drug called *coca-ethylene*. This is then released back into the blood stream. When it hits the brain it gives you another or increased high. Unfortunately, it is highly liver toxic. Not only is it liver toxic but you are likely to be highly grumpy the next day if you then drink or take cocaine on its own, because the brain will think that it is being short changed. It also increases your chances of a heart attack quite dramatically

Similarly, drinking on top of prescribed drugs can range from nullifying their effect to combining themselves into an incredibly strong sedative on the body, sometimes with tragic outcomes.

Drug users cannot take their drugs and then enjoy their 21 units on top. Alcohol and drugs are often mixed to handle the 'ups' and 'downs' of the different effects but at times it is like trying to make sure that the paddling pool is perfectly positioned under the twenty metre diving board. When it is not then there is a problem when you hit the ground and when it is perfectly positioned it is still high risk behaviour.

Drinking with Drug Use:

Psychological balances:

Opiates produce feelings of detachment; alcohol can reduce anxiety and help someone feel more relaxed.

Alcohol can be a replacement drug.

Alcohol allows a process of 'normalisation'; it can enable drug users to feel like they are 'fitting in OK'.

Alcohol can help to minimise the increasing dependence/use of drugs, by blaming the short term effect of excessive alcohol.

Alcohol can often replace some drug use, in what appears to be successful harm reduction drug treatment, or even abstinence from drug use.

Alcohol in addition to drug use will significantly increase liver damage, especially for those who have hepatitis C.

Alcohol on top of the depressive drugs – eg. heroin, tranquilisers, methadone - increases the sedative effects and overdose is common.

Most drug overdoses and drug deaths are alcohol-related.

Related to many of the points above, alcohol mixed with drugs increases the likelihood of poor decision-making and denial of the risk.

Alcohol is strongly related to drug relapse or behaviour relapse. The Howard League has reported over 50 per cent of young offenders re-offended under the influence of alcohol. Alcohol MUST BE SEEN AS A GATEWAY DRUG.

Loss of memory, 'black outs', passing out increases the risk of serious accident or death. Choking on their own vomit is a common cause of death for those with serious alcohol misuse problems.

Medication/prescription drugs

Medical advice should always be sought. Alcohol can negate some medicines (such as antibiotics) but not all. The doctors advice about not drinking when being prescribed antibiotics harks back to the days of treating for VD, where the fear was that drinking was likely to lead to an increased likelihood of sex and sexually transmitted diseases. As you will see from the NHS advice below, there are clear and specific reasons why drinking alcohol with certain antibiotics is ill advised), enhance or suppress effects, or cause serious side-effects (physical and psychological). All good agencies should have a copy of MIM's available or download.

From the NHS Choices web-site

When to avoid drinking alcohol completely
It is necessary to completely avoid drinking alcohol when taking the antibiotics described below.

Metronidazole
Metronidazole is sometimes used to clear dental, or vaginal, infections, or to clear infected leg ulcers, or pressure sores.

Tinidazole
Tinidazole is sometimes used to treat many of the same infections as metronidazole, as well as to help clear bacteria called Helicobacter pylori (H pylori) from the gut.

Drinking alcohol when you are taking either metronidazole, or tinidazole, can cause a serious reaction. The symptoms of this reaction include: breathlessness, headaches, chest pain, skin flushing, increased or irregular heartbeat, low blood pressure (hypertension) and nausea and vomiting.

Co-trimoxazole
Occasionally, co-trimoxazole can cause a similar reaction to that of metronidazole, or tinidazole, if you drink alcohol while you are taking it. However, with co-trimoxazole, the side effects above are very rare, and drinking alcohol in moderation does not normally cause a problem.

Linezolid
If you are taking linezolid, you should avoid drinking alcoholic drinks that contain a substance called tyramine, such as wine, beer, sherry, and lager.

Erythromycin
Drinking alcohol while you are taking erythromycin may make you drowsy. Alcohol can also make erythromycin less effective.

Side effects

It is also important to note that some antibiotics may have a variety of side effects, such as sleepiness and dizziness that might be made worse by drinking alcohol. Alcohol is likely to worsen these effects.

A little bit of history of alcohol and drugs

No doubt discussing the general ignorance of the drug treatment filed to alcohol use and misuse will offend a few. For the record, there are doctors and practitioners who deliver excellent alcohol and drug work, who have specialised knowledge and who are shining examples of what the drug treatment field should be. Sadly, they are on the minority side, and even more so the higher you climb through treatment services management, commissioning and national bodies.

At the management and national delivery level I have had many conversations with senior people across the drug treatment spectrum and not one had ever disagreed with me about the above. However, only two have ever done anything about it. The rest offer platitudes and excuses. The most honest answers I ever received were 'well there's no money in alcohol is there, so why bother?'.

In closing this section I offer the salutary lesson that should be remembered from the NTORS study. It should have a high resonance amongst those I have mentioned – sadly it does not.

One of the statistics from the NTORS study was that a significant number of people who successfully completed their drug treatment found that their drinking substantially increased. Even more worryingly, the majority of these people went on to experience significant alcohol misuse problems. Worse still, they reported that their alcohol use was much more damaging to their health and person than their drug use had ever been. A quote that shall always stay in my mind was from an 'ex drug user' who stated that for years he used drugs but it was 'alcohol that bit him in the bum'.

Interestingly enough, I have been told that in the early days of drug treatment in the late 1960s and early 1970s, it was not unusual at a few of the 'Rehabs' (residential treatment services) for the staff and residents to retire down the local pub on a Friday evening to relax and review the week. Presumably, everyone deserved a pint or two after a difficult week of talking about substance misuse.

Mental Health

Mental health diagnosis is a skill that comes from years of study and practice. This section tries to understand alcohol use and misuse in relation to mental health concerns so that the two are not confused.

Someone described as having mental health problems can cover anything in our general jargon from someone with a high level of anxiety and neurosis, through to depression and schizophrenia. It includes a massive range of symptoms and problems. We have all probably heard all of the above described as 'having a breakdown' at some time or other.

When any of the above also involves drinking then it can be very confusing and difficult to unpick all the dynamics.

How many times are you faced with an individual who is drinking but appears to have mental health problems? What is the alcohol problem and what is the mental health problem? How do you differentiate between them and are they intrinsically linked?

When you try to make a referral, it is often the case that the mental health service will not take the referral because of the drinking and the alcohol service cannot work with the mental health problems. What usually tips the balance is a crisis – the risk of or actual self-harm, threats of violence or an accident.

Here are some key issues to consider:

Mental health

Drinking to excess contributes to stress and emotional distress, which are likely to exhibit as mental health problems.

To the family member or partner trying to understand what is happening can be almost impossible – the drinking is spiralling out of control and the behaviour becoming more extreme.

What to do and what to understand from the clues:

The individual may be drinking to control their feelings. This can range from trying to cope with emotional feelings from stress at work through to loss of a loved one; fear of something, divorce, trauma. Alcohol can be a comfort blanket where the thinking stops. The pain is lost in an alcoholic fog.

Drinking can sometimes help some people to control or stop the voices that they are hearing. Differentiating this from auditory hallucinations, which along with visual hallucinations can be part of the withdrawal effects from alcohol, is absolutely crucial.

Drinking because of depression is a common issue but alcohol is also a depressant. This can result in the situation being considerably worse.

Drinking on top of medication can cause further physical and mental health problems, as described previously. The visual and auditory hallucinations that can often be misdiagnosed as mental health problems can also be attributed to disturbed sleep patterns which of course are common to both alcohol misuse and to some mental health problems. These can be very upsetting for the individual. Some practitioners favour so called sleep therapy through medication because it does help to avoid some of this.

The risk of suicide is likely to be in the forefront of any dual diagnosis. Drinking alcohol is often a reason for not admitting someone into hospital. There is a perspective, that drinking makes the risk of an overdose or self-harming more likely. Admission into a place of safety or with a friend or relative will reduce this risk.

Physical health

Alcohol is a sedative and a pain reliever, whether physical or mental. Many paraplegics have used alcohol as a physical pain reliever.

Drinking alcohol can cause a long list of physical problems. From hangovers to peripheral neuritis (tingling in the fingers, numbness through to rigidity of the limbs – it is where the protective sheaths around the nerve endings are damaged), to liver cirrhosis and accidents. It is linked to cancer of the oesophagus, stomach, pancreas. Alcohol does not directly kill the brain cells, the problem is that chronic drinking causes malabsorption of thiamine and this coupled with the fact that many people who drink chronically eat erratically and poorly. It is the thiamine deficiency that causes the neurological problems. In extreme cases this causes what is known as wet brain, where there is permanent brain damage.

Alcohol is a painkiller. Many paraplegics suffer ongoing pain from their injuries on a permanent basis. Prescribed painkillers reach a threshold and cease to be as effective, requiring either larger doses, or a substitute. As a sporting analogy – alcohol wears the number 12 shirt. In addition, pain killers can produce unpleasant side effects that drinking alcohol can nullify or reduce.

Many physical ailments cause great pain – rheumatoid arthritis as an example. Alcohol can nullify or reduce the pain in the short term.

The tip over point from useful and effective drug to becoming an additional problem is a fine line and varies from person to person. From a third party point of view, there are two paths to go down – firstly, trying to cope with constant pain can illicit great sympathy and sadness and drinking can be seen as a positive behaviour and an understandable behaviour.

'I do not blame them given their circumstances'.

This gives a further green light to the person drinking to carry on and of course makes it harder to address when the tipping point is reached.

The second path is the unsympathetic, frustrated or angry reaction to someone who will not help themselves, who is self-pitying, not facing up to reality and drinking too much. As a carer, trying to work or help someone who is physically dependent on you and drinks too much can be extremely difficult, making their physical care harder.

Physical and mental violence

Alcohol is implicated in 86 per cent of murders.
Alcohol is implicated in 45 per cent of all violent crimes (the victims believed their attackers had been drinking)
Alcohol is involved in 37 per cent of domestic violence cases.
Alcohol in 2007-08, was involved in more than a million crimes in some way
Alcohol is implicated in 30 per cent of child abuse cases.
Alcohol is implicated in 50 per cent of stranger violence.

—Figures taken from the Home Office and Alcohol Concern

The Institute of Alcohol Studies in 2010 produced a Fact Sheet on Alcohol and Crime:

Scale of the Problem

The Police Superintendents have advised that alcohol is present in half of all crime. A 1990 study for the Home Office found that growth in beer consumption was the single most important factor in explaining growth in crimes of violence against the person. Research also shows that high proportions of victims of violent crime are drinking or under the influence of alcohol at the time of their assault.

In an analysis of data drawn from 41 probation areas between 1 April 2004 and 31 March 2005

The Offender Assessment System Data Evaluation and Analysis Team found that:

Over one-third (37 per cent) of offenders had a current problem with alcohol use a similar proportion (37 per cent) had a problem with binge drinking nearly half (47 per cent) had misused alcohol in the past 32 per cent had violent behaviour related to their alcohol use 38 per cent were found to have a criminogenic need relating to alcohol misuse, potentially linked to their risk of reconviction

Research has found that alcohol had been consumed prior to the offence in nearly three-quarters (73 per cent) of domestic violence cases and was a 'feature' in almost two-thirds (62 per cent). Furthermore, almost half (48 per cent) of these convicted domestic violence offenders were alcohol dependent. A minimum of 1 in 5 people arrested by police, test positive for alcohol.

An All Party Group of MPs investigating alcohol and crime was advised by the British Medical Association that alcohol is a factor in:
60-70 per cent of homicides
75 per cent of stabbings
70 per cent of beatings
50 per cent of fights and domestic assaults

In Scotland, a study of Accident & Emergency admissions found that at least 70 per cent of cases of assault were possibly related to alcohol. Most of these assaults happened at the weekend and the majority involved people under 30. On the basis of this study, a minimum of 77 alcohol-related assaults present to emergency departments in Scotland every day.

Alcohol and violence is nothing new – when researching the history there are plenty of anecdotes – I read an article from a newspaper reproduced from the seventeenth century reporting on an argument in the Swan Public House in Tottenham that was taken out onto the green outside where it was settled when one of the two ran his sword through the other, killing him.

In the 1920s 'Glasgow fortnight' in Blackpool (when the factories in Glasgow closed for two weeks and folks went on holiday) often turned violent and alcohol-related fighting would result in fatalities.

Drink was usually given and taken, it was recorded during the shield wall battles of the seventh and eighth centuries.

For any counsellor or group worker out there, running an anger management course or counselling without considering alcohol is like driving a car without petrol.

Intoxication is the excuse – the drink cannot be violent in itself and millions of us drink without being violent. But anyone involved in domestic violence, child abuse, stranger violence, either as victim or perpetrator needs to consider their drinking and their drinking behaviour, even if primarily to dismiss it as factor. It is just too common not to.

Domestic Violence

I return to domestic violence again in this section. Alcohol and domestic violence is a quagmire to tackle:

Victims often drink to cope with the violence or the threat of violence.
Victims drinking and behaviour can lead to the violence.
Perpetrators can drink to be violent, as an excuse or as a reason.
Hitting out can be easier than talking.
Drink can be blamed, rather than a lack of control.

Drinking introduces the factor that is never there in couple counselling; it introduces the unpredictability that turns a tense situation violent, it enhances a misunderstanding, it fuels the anger. It brings the mayhem to volatile situations.

There is no sensible drinking level for violence and probably even less so for domestic violence. Domestic violence may not involve alcohol at all. It may involve a few drinks, it may be after a binge, it may be sporadic or incessant, it may be a pattern. None of it is acceptable and it all needs intervention.

Whatever the factors and components of any domestic violence situation, drinking alcohol has to be considered as a potential causal or related factor. It is likely to be a crucial factor in any cessation or solution.

There is a whole book on this subject in itself. Suffice to say that if it is happening then it needs to be addressed and usually with a third party breaking or at least interrupting the cycle.

IMPLICATIONS FOR SERVICES ACROSS DRUGS, MENTAL AND PHYSICAL HEALTH

Initial conversations and assessment:

Alcohol is very likely to be involved in their overall lifestyle to some degree. Accept it and acknowledge it.

Always screen for a client's drinking in addition to drug use, using a drink diary where, when and why and what type of drinking.

Never ask 'do you drink?' but 'how do you drink?' – you are looking for behaviour changes and effects; relationships between drinking, lifestyle and drug use.

You are screening for risk behaviour and attitudes to an individual's use of alcohol and drugs.

At a formal stage or as a piece of homework, ask them to fill in a diary (24 hour) over about a month.

Take a good drink and drug history (for example – there is an issue relating to alcohol metabolism called MEOS Basically if someone is taking opiates and drinking, then the opiates are metabolised faster).

Two Formal Screening techniques:

AUDIT is a comprehensive alcohol screening tool (a copy is reproduced in the appendices)
FAST is a shortened version of the same tool.

Staff skills and Knowledge

An ability to give basic information on alcohol – effects on the body and brain; risk assessment; basic information on alcohol and drugs; where and how to access further information.

Brief interventions on alcohol – teaching simple tools for cutting down consumption; understanding simple cognitive processes under the influence, risk assessment and management, all delivered using basic motivational interviewing/enhancement techniques.

Detoxification

Alcohol is a dangerous drug to stop using if the individual has developed a physical dependence. It is much more toxic than most other drugs. Drugs may be masking the alcohol dependence, especially methadone.

Medical assessments of dependence and withdrawal management may be required.

What a credible treatment provider should have as management tools

A staff team who can:

Talk about drinking and alcohol use in relation to drugs
Alcohol included in holistic assessment and screening processes
Educate on alcohol use & misuse, effects & access to further information
Brief interventions on alcohol and relapse management techniques
Motivational enhancement skills
An ability to teach risk assessment and management

An environment that:

has good information on alcohol use and misuse models of care/care pathways with alcohol providers delivers good training programmes on alcohol for staff assessment forms and care plans that have space to record drinking and alcohol use; targets for reduction; behaviour change.

CHAPTER NINE

IT'S NOT ROCKET SCIENCE – ADVICE FOR WORKING WITH PEOPLE WHO HAVE PSYCHOLOGICAL OR PHYSICAL DEPENDENCE

What is physical dependence?

Alcohol is a highly addictive drug. Physical dependence is likely at about two bottles of wine, a bottle of spirits and six to eight pints of strong lager a day. Again, it depends on the person's body and organs.

It is not an exact science and varies from person to person. Invariably, the person drinking knows, as do those around them.

Stopping suddenly can bring on nasty physical withdrawals from chronic shaking (referred to as delirium tremors), sweating, panic attacks, auditory or visual hallucinations, racing heart, vomiting and even fitting. It can be highly dangerous and will require medication to assist with controlling them.

The classic description of heroin withdrawals is usually exaggerated. In reality the advice you will receive is that you are going to experience flu like symptoms and muscle cramps. It will be highly unpleasant with plenty of sweating. You are going to feel like shite but you are not going to die. With alcohol withdrawals however, there can be a risk of death in rare cases and the fitting can lead to serious injury. Alcohol is a much nastier drug than heroin to withdraw from.

Medical or nursing assistance is the best option. However, many do successfully withdraw from alcohol by reducing their intake over a few days. It is often seen as the kindest way to withdraw (or dry out) for the body. This process is obviously difficult for professionals to advocate from a medical and insurance point of view but in reality is practised widely and with impressive results.

It is viewed adversely because of the 'one drink, one drunk' attitude of recovery and the fact that anyone who is an alcoholic is only ever one drink away from relapse and the disease of addiction.

It is rarely discussed in books and guides, which just further increases the sense of crisis and isolation in the individual and those around them. There is that horrible sense that change and help cannot be achieved without specialist and medical intervention.

In reality everyone is different with different tolerances. Many people are able to cut down and withdraw for themselves. In my experience, this has been done in all manner of ways. In terms of attempting to withdraw from alcohol oneself then it is always best to seek advice from a GP or an alcohol specialist, so that everyone understands risk, how to help, what to watch for and so forth.

What is psychological dependence?

Psychological addiction is another matter. There is no rule of thumb for the quantity. Psychological dependence obviously goes hand in hand with physical dependence and the role of CBT in working with cognitive processing is an integral part of assisting in equipping the person with overcoming psychological dependence.

Although psychological dependence is intrinsically linked with physical dependence, it can also be completely separate and happen well before any stage of physical dependence.

Psychological dependence is personal. One person can be dependent on having 'a couple' of drinks after work or when they get home, for others it gives them confidence to socialise, someone else would say that they cannot cope without a drink and for others they need to have a drink as soon as they get up. Someone else may need to have a few drinks before they go to bed or sleep with their partners.

Alcohol as a depressant can numb physical or emotional pain. The loss of a loved one can be coped with by drinking.

Interpersonal aspects of psychological dependence (coping with change)

The roles of the drinker and the partner need huge untangling. The drinker determined to stop needs and wants to take on responsibility, to gain respect, to become more pro-active. For years he or she has not done this and the partner has had to cope. They take on the role of victim, angel, the man or woman who has to do everything, take on all the responsibilities from child care to working, to paying the bills, to clearing up the vomit and the soiled clothes.

Suddenly everything is changing and even the non-drinking partner has to be stripped of their angel role, give up responsibility, learn to trust and give up control to someone who has had a career of being unreliable.

It is a hell of a change and will need talking about. I have taken a man home from a treatment unit and found a bottle of whisky on the kitchen table from their wife as a 'welcome home' present. Better to sabotage, than face up to change.

The drinker may not have been violent at all but a lovely person who would not harm a fly, never argue but drink. Everyone found him funny or generous. Another drinker may be exciting to be with, a risk taker.

Take away the drink and the partner finds them dull, not the person they met. Taking away the drink can wreck a marriage just as much as drinking can wreck a marriage. Was it the drinking? Was it the relationship? Whatever the answer, you can bet it is the drinking that cops the blame, then the drinker.

The point is that so much needs to change – not only the drinking but the thinking and the behaviour and the environment and the people around them.

Tips for cutting down with dependency

Try to push back that first drink of the day – do not leave the can besides the bed, put it in the fridge (at least it will not be warm and you are on your feet before you have a drink).

Stay in bed when you first wake up.

Brush your teeth (this might sound stupid but it will freshen up your mouth and make the drink taste different).

Try and make a cup of tea as the first drink of the day (it will hydrate you and it is not alcohol pouring down your throat as the first drink of the day).

If you start to manage the above, then next up try and have a bath or shower before your first drink.

Then add additional things – make some toast, take a little exercise, even a few stretches, put the TV or radio on, go outside and take in some fresh air, go and buy a newspaper (basically anything that you think is constructive rather than have that first drink). Then try to extend by five minutes each morning before having that first drink of the day.

Switch drinking from a strong lager or spirit to a weaker beer. When you switch to a weaker lager drink the same amount of volume, or even increase it if you need to and then try to cut it down (and you will be taking in less alcohol).

Try and space the cans.

When you go to the supermarket, the pub or off licence, take a slightly longer route, take a scenic route or a more interesting route.

Start paying attention to personal hygiene and take a bit of time pampering yourself.

Try drinking water or tea and coffee in between drinking a can or wine or spirits.

Force yourself to eat.

Reward yourself with treats.

If you are making progress use the old adage of 'don't get hungry, thirsty or tired' – they all impact on your drinking. Give yourself some goals – write to someone or try and ring someone, seek some non-drinking company, watch something you are interested on the TV.

Sip instead of gulping.

The aim of these tactics is to cut down to a level that you feel comfortable with. You are doing it for yourself, so you set the goals. Should you want to push on then only you can decide. No one is going to persuade you or tell you.

Should you continue along these lines then sometime between 3 and 10 days, then your body will be completely alcohol free.

This will feel strange indeed and quite contradictory. On the one hand you are likely to feel physically much better and optimistic but on the other hand scared to have a drink and then screaming for a drink or just tempted to have a drink. There may even be a little voice in your head that suggests that perhaps you were not really dependent (or an alcoholic).

This is when you need to build on it and to talk with others (expert or not) so that these sensations, feelings and thoughts can be talked about and let out into the open for you to look at and understand and so that you can begin to enjoy the new relationship that you are going to have with your body and a sober you.

CHAPTER TEN

IT'S NOT ROCKET SCIENCE – ADVICE FOR YOUNG PEOPLE AND YOUNG ADULTS

Firstly, what do we mean by young people?

There is an important distinction between those who are under eighteen (young people) and those between eighteen and twenty five (young adults).

Why the distinction?

It is illegal to sell alcohol to anybody under the age of eighteen. In reality, 80 per cent of that group are going to drink alcohol, some of them from the age of ten but most will experiment with alcohol on numerous occasions between fifteen and eighteen.

For everyone over eighteen and under twenty five they are legally entitled to drink, have varying income available to drink, have a limited amount of options to socialise elsewhere than where drink is available and are from a group heavily targeted by the wider drinks industry. These factors combined lend themselves to the drinking culture that our city centres 'enjoy' almost as a nightly experience. They are therefore incredibly vulnerable.

There is also another very important factor why I make a distinction. We often talk about the changes that teenagers go through with their physical and hormonal changes, the changes in mood, learning to stand on their own two feet and so forth.

These changes on the whole take place against a background of some form of parental home, school or college and of course peer pressure.

Personally, I think that individuals go through greater change between eighteen and twenty five. They are forced to be increasingly independent both emotionally and financially. It is often the beginning of regular work and education outside of school. Romance and relationships with peers take on a more serious side and individuals appear to undergo a greater introspection and consciousness.

Individual's handwriting and signatures change, their appearance often changes. For some, the arrival of children – planned or unplanned – occurs.

There is a financial independence of sorts, although escaping the family home appears to be increasingly difficult in the current economic climate.

All this is happening as you start to drink legally. Learning how to drink and handle yourself is a real learning curve. Alcohol, as we have been discussing, is a powerful sedative that unlocks the brain in all sorts of ways – not only in terms of mechanical control but emotionally. At this age, most of us are beginning to form a relationship with alcohol, for better and for worse and in sickness and in health.

Even more so now is the lack of alternative venues to socialise in. Of course there is the church or the gym or the local Starbucks, but 90 per cent of eighteen to twenty five year olds are going to choose the pub or club because that's where their mates are, that's where you will meet the opposite sex and that's where all the fun is.

So there you are that is why I make such a serious distinction. I think that the period between eighteen and twenty five is pretty perilous for everyone. In relation to drinking alcohol it is where pretty firm behaviours are learnt and can become entrenched because of patterns of behaviour and labels that tend to stick with individuals.

Young people

Drinking alcohol is a legal option for everyone over eighteen. You cannot expect anyone to abstain from something and then suddenly at eighteen start drinking with no repercussions. That makes no sense at all and could even be seen as a dangerous and irresponsible attitude but that technically is the current situation.

This book argues that it is the duty of all responsible adults to properly prepare young people for such a dangerous drug as alcohol. However, we are hardly in a good position to be responsible adults to young people and young adults.

As a nation we have an ambiguity about our drinking. On the whole we enjoy our drinking. As has been made clear, drinking relaxes us and helps make us laugh. It can make us feel more confident. A couple of drinks and we all think we may be a little thinner, all a little sexier or handsome, better company, less stressed, we can be amusing. Going to the pub makes life seem better.

Yet nearly everyone has had an experience that we would define as negative around alcohol from making ourselves feel ill, having an accident through to being loose tongued, argumentative, verbally violent and even physically violent.

We may have behaved embarrassingly, or done something that we later regretted.

All in all, it's a real double edged sword and takes a few years to get the balance right (some of us never do!).

Overlay this with religious and moral beliefs around not drinking and the taboos that are associated with this and we have an even more complicated situation.

So, it is not surprising then that how we introduce young people to alcohol is confused and often unclear. We do this at a strategic level through the government whether through public health, criminal justice, licensing. We do it as adults and we do it as parents. Young people see us drink as parents and adults and make their own minds up from mimicking, to disgust, to excuse and reason. They watch our moods change, our unpredictability.

As is constantly stated, it is a legal substance, our social occasions and festivals revolve around drinking, we see the adverts in newspapers and magazines, on the TV, in our supermarkets and shops.

Most of us try to introduce our off-spring to alcoholic beverages as a treat or as a way of acknowledging that they are growing up. We cannot buy them a drink until they are eighteen but we can for a party at home or in a pub with a meal or on holiday.

We know that they are going to experiment with drink; most of us consider drinking as a better alternative to taking 'drugs' though not necessarily depending on circumstances. We know our influence as parents is strong but limited and that at times, peers are going to have a much greater influence.

There is no special strategy for young adults and there is certainly no proper strategy, nor preparation for young people. Young people are banned from drinking. They can drink with a meal in a restaurant but there is no real guidance for parents and responsible adults. In this way, we take a risk with what we think might be practical.

At parties a blind eye is turned as teenagers 'mine sweep' or raid the fridge and drink in the garden or a bedroom. Some adults will be strict and some will allow their children to have one bottle of beer but are usually uncomfortable about what to say to their own children's friends.

There is no advice or help for parents. Alcohol is discussed in schools as part of the curriculum but it is flimsy to say the least and is never treated by the teachers and the Department of Education like illegal drugs are.

Young adults

At times, for those over eighteen and living at home, it will seem that to parents their whole world revolves around going out and drinking. What money they do earn is never seen in the house apart from music and clothes. The proportion of money spent on alcohol and going out (drinking alcohol) for many will take up to 80 per cent of their weekly income.

For many this is where their relationship with drink starts to be formed.

The drinks industry in their drink awareness campaigns very much capture the issues and 'hit the nail on the head' but these appear to fail to influence behaviour.

Why this happens has to be understood in the context of the environment, the peer pressure, the expectation of alcohol equals fun and irresponsibility, the promotional campaigns of the venues and the most important fact:

Alcohol is a drug and intoxicant. It alters cognitive processes. It blurs reality and thinking. An advert on the TV, sober and in a bedroom or living room makes complete sense. After two or three drinks the message is ineffective and immaterial.

It is this area that the licensed premises need to take an incredibly strong role as lead educator and harm reductionists. Not information about units but from the ground upwards in terms of design of the buildings, seating, music ambience and about behaviour. Door staff who are there to ensure that inside is orderly and safe (yet fun), no entry after 10.30 pm (say) and applying all the issues as covered under the management of licensed premises.

As has been said, between the age of eighteen and twenty five individuals go through enormous emotional change and huge steps in lifestyle from education to employment (or unemployment), from home to independent living, trying out new living arrangements, legal adult entertainment, mobility through cars and bikes, no responsibilities to big responsibilities, more disposable income than ever before.

Yes, we know all this, I hear you say, but what about the drinking? Well everything always needs to be considered in context.

YOUNG ADULTS AND ALCOHOL SUGGESTIONS

Do not label anyone's drinking behaviour for young adults.

Do not use terms like dependency, binge drinking or any other label.

Discuss the drinking for what it is – if it is becoming a pattern or a prop or a problem in terms of behaviour then it needs to be talked about. The behaviour may elicit all sorts of emotional reactions but the drinking needs to be discussed like we would drugs – where is it harmful and where is it safe? Can it be reduced? Can the harmful effects tackled?

Try to have two or three days not drinking.

Apply the tactics laid out in basic information.

No alcohol when driving or leave the car at home – serious.

Look at expenditure on drinking against income. This is always an interesting exercise as it can be very illuminating.

Look at drinking impact on lifestyle.

What does everyone else see when you are drunk? Funny and handsome or tiresome and ugly?

Are you missing any days at work or is your performance at work suffering? Is it noticed?

Have you lost things like mobile phones, wallets, handbag, and money when you have been out drinking? Why is this?

What about fights and arguments? Is your drinking involved?

What about STDs and Pregnancy. Is drinking involved?

It is a bloody mine field learning to drink. It should be fun and involve happy times of laughter, friendship and love. It really should, and if it is not then something is wrong and needs to be addressed or at least toned down.

THE LEGAL SITUATION

It is worth reminding readers about what the law is in the UK with regards to drinking ages. The following was written by the Chief Medical Officer and was agreed in 2009. It appears on the Drink Aware web-site (www.drinkaware.co.uk):

Official UK Government Guidelines on Drinking Under the Minimum Legal Drinking Age of 18

The British government has published official government advice for young people and their parents about drinking alcohol. The government recommends that:

- *Children should not drink before they're 15, if at all.*
- *5 to 17-years-olds should only drink when they're supervised by a parent or other adult.*
- *If 15 to 17-year-olds drink, they should do so infrequently and definitely on no more than one day a week. Parents*

> *and young people should be aware that drinking, even at 15 or older, can be dangerous to health. Not drinking is the healthiest option for young people.*

- *The importance of parents' influence on their children's drinking should be made clear. Parents and carers need advice on how to respond to alcohol use and misuse by children.*
- *Support services must be available for young people who have alcohol-related problems and to their parents.*

The government emphasizes that this advice is based on the research conducted by a panel of experts.

Young persons between the ages of seven and 17 are legally able to drink alcoholic beverages with parental or guardian consent.

So in a nutshell, you can buy alcohol over the age of 18 and give it to your five year old son and daughter. Yes, that is correct—technically you can give your five year old son a can of Stella or Bud and watch football sponsored by Carlsberg (along with others). It states nothing about supervised consumption. Please note that there is a bland and meaningless sentence 'Children should not drink before they're 15, if at all'.

I will leave you to make up your own mind about this — on one level you can argue that it is good healthy libertarian stuff; on another level, given what we know about the damage alcohol can cause, it could be argued that this is irresponsible. Suffice to say, if this was a work of fiction you wouldn't make it up.

CHAPTER ELEVEN

TOOLS OF THE TRADE

Drink Diaries

Drink Diaries may sound pedantic but countless numbers of people have found them useful and say so. Simply writing down when, why and where they drank is a really useful tool to review and understand one's drinking behaviour.

A diary simply keeps a retrospective account of your drinking – when, where and how much you spent. When you go through it, then why you drink when you did and how you felt during it and after it are interesting and often self-revelatory to the diary keeper.

You see the penny drop for individuals as they look back and see the patterns and the private realisations of their behaviour.

Some are appalled at the cost of their drinking. Others can understand their relationship difficulties. They are a really invaluable tool both for the individual concerned but also the professional, as there before you is all the material to work with in front of you, written down by that person.

Detoxification

This book has tried to look at the process of reducing the harm and cutting down on one's drinking. For some, the more radical approach of stopping altogether may be necessary.

Stopping altogether has to be done carefully, as the potential withdrawal effects can be dangerous and in some cases life threatening.

Withdrawing from alcohol will cause a range of physical and psychological effects depending on the level of physical dependency, personal health and circumstances.

The effects as described previously for alcohol withdrawal include in the milder form sweating, shaking, heart racing, auditory and visual hallucinations, anxiety and panic, through to the danger of alcohol-related fitting and in rare cases heart failure.

It is not a pleasant experience and as such is a powerful catalyst in the person for not wanting to stop.

Some individuals will choose to cut down their drinking over a few days or a week or ten days and stopping thus giving themselves a self-detoxification. This process is not without risk but in one aspect allows the body to reduce its demands and cravings for the drug – alcohol. Just stopping drinking is not advised as this can lead to the very severe end of the symptoms described above and on rare occasions can lead to grave complications and even death.

For the majority, the best process is to seek a detoxification through medication either supervised through a GP, nurse or Alcohol Treatment Programme, or in a specialist unit or hospital.

The main issues to contemplate are where the person feels safest and can be supported, where they can sleep (because sleep patterns during dependent drinking will be badly disturbed and many of the vision and auditory hallucinations are likely to be related to sleep deprivation rather than the drinking). However, alcohol inhibits GABA, so when you stop drinking then GABA becomes excited and stimulates the brain. This is cited as another reason for these hallucinations. After 30 years of talking and working with experts and also carrying out a trawl of the internet, I am, to be honest still unclear on the cause. Both make some sense to me.

But while we are on the subject - what is GABA, I hear you ask?

GABA, or gamma-aminobutyric acid, is the most abundant inhibitory neurotransmitter in the brain. While GABA is an amino acid, it is classified as a neurotransmitter and helps induce relaxation and sleep. It balances the brain by inhibiting over-excitation. GABA contributes to motor control, vision, and many other cortical functions. Anxiety is also regulated by GABA. Some drugs that increase the level of GABA in the brain are used to treat epilepsy and to calm the trembling of people suffering from Huntington's disease.

Medical services have a range of drugs that they use to assist with the withdrawals and compliment these with additional vitamins. They will encourage you to drink lots of water and tea to help the liver flush out the toxins.

Self Help

This manual is designed for self-help and to assist anyone to help you – be they a relative, friend, colleague or a professional.

The best self-help organisation in the world is Alcoholics Anonymous (AA). Many advocates of AA would strongly disagree about many of the approaches in this book, because they are strong advocates of alcoholism being a disease or an illness.

AA is available as a group or individual support in every town in the UK. They will never turn you away (unless you are violent to them). They will listen and will talk. It is free, it is anonymous and many friends and colleagues consider that it has saved their lives, which is good enough for me.

Their contact details are on the Internet, in Yellow Pages, local newspapers, in libraries, NHS services and at police stations. They are not in the public houses and off licences (and they bloody well should be, but we will come to that in the last chapter).

My favourite quote from a member of Alcoholics Anonymous, is when someone says 'I tried AA and did not like it'. To which comes the reply: 'And how many times have you tried a drink?'

They are respectful and supportive whilst at the same time hard-nosed and long in the tooth to counter any smart arse I have ever met with an excuse to carry on drinking.

There are a number of off shoots of AA – Al Anon is for partners, family and friends; Al Ateen is for children of drinkers. They are free and open to anyone.

One of the interesting important aspects of AA is not just the meetings but the fact that anyone can have a sponsor. A sponsor is someone who you can have as a personal contact. They are someone you feel safe with, who might accompany you to see the doctor, who you can phone up if you are feeling like taking a drink or are upset or worried; who will take you to a meeting.

The people at AA are guided by a set of rules, which they refer to as the 12 steps. The first of these is admitting that you are powerless over alcohol. The steps take you through a process of gaining control and responsibility over your life, with you eventually having the opportunity to be a sponsor of someone who is at that first step.

It is a really powerful process for many. It does not suit everyone but it is without doubt the most effective self-help group in the world and should never be discounted lightly.

Brief Interventions, Counselling and Group work

In previous chapters, concepts and approaches about Cognitive Behavioural Treatment and the Cycle of Change were mentioned.

These approaches, through Brief Interventions, Counselling, Therapy and Group Work form the basis for the majority of programmes offering treatment for individuals.

The simple ones teaching relapse management and prevention focus on how our brains work. The counselling and therapy work tends to focus more on underlying emotional/self/family issues and considering your drinking as a response to these (or vice versa). Then there are more deep rooted therapies such as Transactional Analysis, where you are to use their terms 'peeling away the layers of onion skins' in order to look deeper into who you are in order to understand your drives, aspirations and fears.

The bottom line for me – is to learn to walk before you run. Cut down and give yourself credit, stop if you want or need to and give yourself credit. Give yourself time to feel and function without being reliant or dominated by alcohol and give yourself credit.

Start to tackle the immediate problems and give yourself credit, start to make amends to damaged relationships and give yourself credit.

In AA the talk is about one day at a time and a host of other truisms. Truisms work, because they are truisms and have been tried and tested by many people over much time.

Abstinence (stopping) vs. Harm Reduction (reducing the harm)

Abstinence and Harm Reduction are not separate things. They are often made out to be but they are not, especially when they are considered on a continuum. Both involve reducing the harm and the desired outcome of either will only work with the desire and willingness of the individual. We can, as professionals and family, give all the best advice and pressure them but it will not make a scrap of difference. Doctors can fill someone up with a drug that stops them drinking in the short term but when it runs out, if the desire for change is not there then the drinking will simply recommence, often at an even more damaging way.

Individuals will show a desire to change or they will become sick of their lifestyle or just plain sick and the need or desire to change will formulate, sometimes fleetingly, sometimes more solidly. How we react and handle this can make a difference. What they do not need is someone telling them they have to be abstinent or to try harm reduction.

Lately, there has been a term that has crept into the vocabulary in the form of 'recovery' and it has sparked considerable discussion. For many the term recovery is viewed as recovering from addiction by becoming abstinent and has been greatly ambushed by those who advocate abstinence over harm reduction.

In the mental health field, the term 'recovery' is what the user deems it to be. That will do for me. As has already been stated, there can be no abstinence without harm reduction and abstinence usually happens after considerable attempts at reducing the harm have not produced the desired outcomes. Abstinence is probably the most extreme form of harm reduction and what is important throughout this entire process is the individual feeling that they are gaining control over their own lives and emotions.

Relapse Prevention

I have included a short piece on relapse prevention because it is important. Relapse prevention is basically about not returning to old thinking, which will exhibit themselves as familiar habits and attitudes.

Part of any process of changing behaviour is that it is unlikely that the changes you desire may happen overnight but that in reality you will find that it is a longer process. In terms of drinking, people will stop or cut down and then find they are returning to old behaviours and then cutting down or stopping again.

It is the degree of concern that relapse behaviour has on the individual and those around him/her that more often causes the damage. For example, someone who acknowledges that they can no longer drink and stop, starts a programme or goes to AA meetings and then relapses. They feel they have failed. This can be reinforced by family and friends who feel that the person cannot be trusted. How family and friends react, can trigger a crisis rather than just a simple relapse.

There is much work on how much the individual drinker can manipulate everyone around them to over react and to be rejected and criticised, as an excuse or justification to drink further, to disappear off as worthless or in anger and for those feelings to feed their drinking.

How your brain works its emotions and comes to terms with changes in chemical levels, how it learns to cope with stress or conflict or loss or sadness without its usual dependent drug is really the key to being able to manage change.

I have listened to people talking about being cocooned in alcohol (and a heroin user described their use as at times being like wrapped up in a big duvet where it is warm and you cannot see or hear anyone). Unfortunately, like any drug, alcohol becomes less and less effective at creating this embrace.

Overcoming a dependency usually involves a process of stopping (or cutting down), a relapse and a return to stopping (or cutting down). The normal pattern is for the periods of sobriety or control to become longer and longer and the relapses shorter and less severe (barring accidents), almost like a fire slowly burning out.

In the periods of sobriety and control, this is when constructive changes can be made by the individual as they seek to take control over parts of their lives and to start to earn some trust from partners and families that they can be responsible to take some control (which usually involves then giving up some control and having to trust, which of course can be tortuous and a minefield).

As thinking changes, so there are step changes. I have listened to people saying that their old lifestyle had become boring, that there was more to life, that physically they could not do it anymore. These are all constructs within our thinking (cognition) that are designed to reinforce our positive behaviour at the expense of our previous negative behaviour.

It is what the trade calls 'cognitive dissonance'. For any of us to indulge in behaviour that we know is wrong we need to build excuses or barriers. If it is an affair then usually they need to be hidden, if it is as simple as staying down the pub then the phone died or I did not realise the time or a friend was depressed – never a quick phone call to say that I am going to be an hour late, I hope that is OK.

Someone who smokes cigarettes and knows they should stop will talk about cutting down, or smoking lighter cigarettes. Earlier defences would have been that I am young and will eventually stop or who wants to live forever, or I need to smoke with the stress at work. You will find any defence that lessens the argument in the head (the dissonance), even if you know that it is not entirely true.

Parallel to this is the unlearning of the positives of drinking or the acceptance that drinking no longer brings the positives.

As has been described previously, we all have experiences of happy times drinking, really positive times of drinking that were fun, outrageous, led to meeting people, reinforced you as an individual, led to sex, took risks and so forth.

Against this we have a long list of embarrassing times, of accidents of being ill or behaving badly, of being violent and so forth.

The brain's job is to promote the good experiences and to remember them and talk about them and to try to nullify and bury the bad experiences. It is often not until someone has started their long journey into sobriety that these painful memories are remembered and sometimes need to be tackled with loved ones.

Individuals and their loved ones almost need to come to a 'compact or agreement' on what has to be dumped into the dustbin of history in order for everyone to move forward and what has to be said, apologised for and then also move on. There is often a lot to do but it can be very simple and straightforward if everyone tries.

If this can happen then a relapse can be viewed as a very brief interruption in the context of stopping or cutting down. Personally, I think that relapse can be very intuitive and a positive experience, as it can quicken up the overall change process, especially as most relapses tend to reinforce the need for change.

Unfortunately, it is not something to promote, especially where you have the prevailing belief that in recovery, you are only one drink away from relapse and disaster. When in reality, no one alcoholic drink is responsible for setting off such mayhem and addiction – it is the person who has been building and planning to drink and by hook or by crook, they will do their best to engineer a situation where they can justify a drink.

So what is relapse prevention?

Relapse prevention is all about understanding how your thinking and emotions function and how we can guard against returning to old behaviours. It is about coming to understand that the days we wake up tired and grumpy are natural to us all and not because you are an alcoholic or dependent drinker and need a drink. It is about understanding that maybe you need to alter your route home after work because you have to walk past the pub where you always stopped in for 'one or two', or possibly when you are stronger walking past that same pub with your family and feeling good about yourself because you no longer drink.

It is about understanding how our memories work and that smells and tastes can suddenly catch us unawares and are associated with past experiences involved in drinking. A song on the radio unexpectedly casts you back into a party you were at where something happened or where you met someone you ended up falling in love with and you wonder what happened to them and what went wrong with your life and suddenly you are having a bad day and feeling overwhelmed with emotion and want to have a drink.

Relapse prevention is about accepting that this is normal and you need to take away the urges physically first – make a cup of tea, go and eat something, talk to someone – anything that takes away those initial thoughts, and then explore those thoughts carefully and weigh them up.

Relapse prevention is about understanding the control that you have over your own life and that, at the beginning, you are learning to constantly adjust because you are unlearning learnt behaviour.

On one level, how the brain works and our cognitive processes operate sounds complicated but in essence it is pretty simple, especially if you understand that we as humans operate at all sorts of emotional and physical levels and that words and language have been designed only to articulate those feelings and emotions. It is why things like hugs, walking, sport and stroking the cat probably all work better than sitting in a group therapy session for some.

Though having said that, you will need to find someone you can trust to talk with. You need to find someone who you can check things out with, someone who is on your wave length and understands your drives. In AA, the whole idea of a sponsor or buddy works really well.

Alternatively, it can be a professional counsellor or a friend or family member. You can choose the setting and the place. I do not promote this idea because I do not know enough about it but there are people who do this via the internet and therefore never know the other person or group.

Whatever, it is about finding someone who you can explore your thought processes with and to risk assessing for the future.

Some practical thoughts

I have tried to run through the rudiments of various interventions that are available or little shifts each of us can make to change our behaviour in small ways.

I have also had the privilege of sitting and listening to a whole host of wonderful people talking about their drinking, or someone else's, their problems and how they changed their lives. I have listened to a range of professionals and friends and want to take this opportunity to bring together this pooled thinking on what else is important but never gets mentioned or has been ironed out by either the misery of dependent drinking or by professional and policy makers who always think that they know best.

So here are a few thoughts:

Physical Contact

Many people who have developed serious drinking problems are often quite isolated, not only emotionally but physically. When I first started working in a busy drop in centre in Kings Cross in London, I worked with a wonderful woman called Gladys. Gladys described herself as a recovering alcoholic and was a largish Welsh lady with what I can only describe as an ample chest.

Now Gladys was someone who everyone was drawn to and she would simply hug people when she met them and when they departed, when they were crying or sad and sit close to them when they were talking, but she also kept her distance if she thought that was what someone wanted. The serenity, smiles and happiness that came over many of the men (who attended the drop in) when they were hugged by Gladys was actually very special. It was not remotely sexual.

These men were often existing on the streets, had lost family and friends and a lot of their self-respect and a hug from Gladys was better therapy than any counsellor I have seen in action. She was advised by managers that this behaviour lacked professional boundaries and she would question that and ask what sort of professionals constructed such boundaries in the first place.

I am not suggesting that we always go around hugging everyone but I am suggesting that many professionals and their services create very sterile atmospheres for people who have probably slept alone for years and who have lacked any physical closeness never mind intimacy for years. Stopping and cutting down on drinking, or admitting faults and wrong doing is a highly emotional experience.

Physical Exercise

On one level, I am writing about the blindingly obvious but on another level the issue is not mentioned within the drug treatment strategy and does not form part of any commissioning strategy across health and local authorities.

In assisting anyone to overcome an alcohol (or drug) problem we are trying to develop a new and different lifestyle away from alcohol. We are trying to encourage an individual to go for a walk, to go swimming or to the gym as an alternative to sitting on the sofa at home drinking or going to the pub. This will also provide an opportunity to meet new people away from a drinking environment.

On another level we are trying to encourage physical exercise because of the effect. Drinking is a pretty idle pastime and exercise forces an individual to burn up calories and to become more active. There is much research that points to physical exercise affecting brain chemical (endorphin) activity. Simply put, physical activity will help anyone feel a little better about them, improving self-esteem, to feel healthier and fitter.

For me it raises huge questions about re-assessing what we spend money on in relation to some alcohol and drug treatment. The benefits of a monthly gym or swimming pool pass may well outweigh a weekly counselling session.

I am not aware that there is much research on these types of comparison because the existing treatment providers would not countenance seeing their budgets for services disappear in this way.

Terminology

The last few paragraphs are a timely reminder about terminology. The first part of the book pointed out the need to be very careful with terminology as it was a key to creating successful change.

Here's a few – Alcoholic, Social Drinker, Drunkard, Bum, Abstinent, Recovering alcoholic, Heavy Drinker, Teetotaller, Dipsomania, Vagrant, Street Drinker, Public Drinker, Barfly.

Which label do you want?

How do you explain yourself to people when stopping or cutting down? Take a label from above and explain your circumstances?

My name is Tony and I am an alcoholic!

How about – 'I'd love a cup of tea or coffee', 'I don't fancy a drink', or 'I don't drink'.

Throw the labels out, keep to your own language.

AA talk about 'keeping it simple'. It is one of life's great messages whatever we do. Life is simple but we constantly make it complicated.

Everyone has a forename and a surname, deserves respect and has a story to tell. If they are experiencing difficulties with their drinking whatever the angle, this is how they need to be listened to and afforded help and advice – they do not need a label as a further burden.

In closing

Most of mankind has drank alcohol from the mists of time, from fermenting fruit to home brewed concoctions to buying it in a bar. Whatever religion governs – it is there legally or illegally. Man's ingenuity means it is distilled in prisons, made at home or marketed and sold ('pushed') in quantities that make the illegal drugs trade look like small fry.

Legally it is marketed in a variety of products. Spirits, beer and wine are the three main categories but underneath each of these categories are products that are rich and varied, are all uniquely marketed and sold, to which we all develop attachments and likings, loyalty and preferences.

The tax and duty on the sale of alcohol makes governments around the world billions and billions of pounds, dollars, euros, shekels, yen, rand and so forth. In the UK this figure is around £14 billion.

The cost of alcohol misuse runs into the billions as well but is not quite accounted for in the same way. The good thing for government is that excess alcohol does affect the health of some and substantially reduces life expectancy for this group. This of course reduces overall cost to government. They die younger avoiding pension and expensive social and health care costs. This is a very cynical view I know but one that must factor into our thinking somewhere along the line.

When you find your own drinking has become a concern or a full blown problem, if drinking has caused consequences, then you might have a sympathetic ear or two to start with but structurally the drinking is your fault and your problem. You are on your own. There are services available but they are limited.

Because you are more or less on your own then I hope the last few chapters help and Good Luck.

PART 3

CHAPTER TWELVE

WHAT TO DO WITH THIS MESS?

There can be no doubt that the United Kingdom has a major problem with alcohol. This problem is with the way in which a substantial segment of the population drink and with the behaviour of a significant majority when under the influence of alcohol.

This is seen through alcohol-related ill health and physical harm, through physical and verbal violence, disorder and disturbance.

Clearly there are groups of people who are at risk from alcohol, or more susceptible than others.

Unfortunately, these people are all lumped in with the general population approach of public health. This general population approach looks at overall consumption. The belief of this approach is that if you reduce overall consumption then overall harms come down. You affect overall consumption by dampening demand by increasing prices or you restrict overall supply.

I have likened this approach and others of the last thirty years to re-arranging the deckchairs on the Titanic. Every re-arrangement is accompanied by tough talking Ministers, who like to tell us that they take alcohol seriously and intend to bring about change.

The problem I have is that I have heard a succession of them say exactly the same and move on having done nothing. They simply come with their rhetoric, then see alcohol as a hot potato and go. They stand up at conferences, make a speech and go. They never listen to the other speakers but are generous enough to take a couple of questions and go. They sit in on TV and radio interviews, say a few bland things and go.

The long game means that the problem just becomes worse.

There is a second dynamic that causes as much damage as the political intransigence, possibly more. Previous pages have reflected on the continual argument between the broader 'alcohol industry' and public and national health along with the alcohol lobbyists. This is the fallout from the lack of any commitments or strategic thinking from any government.

Within Public and National Health and the Voluntary Sector (once referred to as the charitable sector) there is a view that the alcohol industry cannot be trusted and is akin to the devil. Their money should not be touched, as it is tainted. It is the same for tobacco. It has been my experience that this position is quoted by many in the sector. It is a rather superior and opinionated position that very much takes the higher moral ground, but is a commonly expressed opinion.

It is a very blinkered viewpoint but one that achieves nothing whilst alleviating the person or organisation holding that point of view from any responsibility to do something.

There is a reality that every voluntary sector organisation, NHS service, public health department, every school and education department, all law and order services and every town hall service, take money from the government coffers. This list includes every ministry and department. It extends to every one of these employees.

In order to fund these services and jobs, the government raises taxes and duties. A significant part of this income is the £14 billion from the tax and duty on alcohol and over £6 billion from the sale of tobacco products. On top of this is corporation tax paid by the companies who produce the alcohol, by the off licences and supermarkets who sell the drinks and the licensed premises of bars, public houses, clubs and restaurants who also sell it. Finally there is the workforce of the above who pay income tax. It is a very sizeable sum.

This income is raised from legal products produced by legal companies with shareholders. We all know that. It is implicit in the fabric and structure of our society. Therefore, part of the government funding to the NHS, to our schools to our voluntary sector is implicitly based on income sourced from alcohol and tobacco. People choose to forget this.

When I raise this issue with senior managers in Drug Treatment and International NGOs, with Consultants in Public Health, they will not accept the link and even if they do, certainly will not forfeit the money which, by their own argument, is tainted.

Whether this is a valid argument or a side issue, the important dynamic is that those who should be in a position to enter into dialogue and constructive debate choose not to and sit back on their moral and ethical position that to talk with the industry is wrong for no better reason than because they are basically 'untrustworthy and evil'.

What is even worse from my point of view is that most of these individuals, who I am criticising for their stance, are quite happy to go and have a beer or two (or even stagger around drunk at conference functions).

'I'll take their money as long as it washed first by the government, I'll drink their products, sometimes to the point of being drunk but I won't talk to them or listen to them'.

That is a quote from me during a rant in 2011. Again, you could not really make it up could you? At least when you read the chapter on the history of alcohol, people like Joseph Livesey and the Temperance Movement led by example and took the pledge themselves. The modern day moralists are not even worthy of the consideration of equivalence.

I will give you an excellent example of this. This is my understanding of how discussions went. Two years ago, I was tasked with raising funds through sponsorship for an International Conference. A tobacco company wanted to participate and support the conference, but the worry for the organisers was that this would not be acceptable to the World Health Organisation and that 'tobacco companies are dodgy' – his solution was to accept the money if they paid for delegate places but they could not sponsor the conference because it would cause problems.

I was actually quite shocked by this and refused to discuss this further. I was being asked to funnel money in through the back door whilst maintaining a front door stance that this very moral and righteous NGO did not accept tobacco money, for no other reason than he and his board felt they were dodgy and that it would upset International Organisations.

They also reversed a decision and ceased taking funding from an international drinks company on the grounds that they cannot buy their way into a conference.

So, if there is to be a change in this intransigence, then there needs to be some major changes across the board. Firstly, it will need to involve those who have not appointed themselves as our moral arbiters.

My proposal would be to ask the people of the United Kingdom what they think. What do we all really think about alcohol in our society? What do we think about our drinking? What do we really think about our city centres and the availability of alcohol? Has any politician ever asked us? Has there ever been an informed national debate rather than a few ramblings in the House of Commons or Lords or in a few weekly radio 'phone in' programmes?

There needs to be a far reaching, informed debate on our attitudes and beliefs to alcohol. The only role our politicians should have in the debate is to explain why they have been so ineffective over the last thirty years, why they have struggled with alcohol compared with say drugs, HIV and AIDS, mental health, domestic violence and heart disease. The politician's role, I would suggest, is to listen and to understand what their future duties will be in relation to alcohol.

This is not some stupid referendum, with an ambiguous question that is specially designed to confuse and cloud the issue, so that is becomes meaningless.

Only then can we start to frame our future society and culture in relation to our drinking behaviour.

In order to make this an informed debate, we will need to have the facts in front of us.

Research

On the issue of alcohol we need to be clear about what we know already and what we still need to know. We also need to learn from what happened with the Drugs Strategy.

Much of the funding for the drugs strategy was the result of research which made the link between drug use and crime – principally heroin and the crime committed by those who were physically addicted to heroin in order to feed their habit. The level of this crime was, according to the research, enormous and the Labour government under Tony Blair saw this as a massive opportunity to significantly reduce overall crime.

Indeed such was the supposed connection that once the first 100,000 heroin users were locked into treatment and monitored and, we were being told, successfully treated, then the national crime rate should have nose-dived. This did not happen.

The two questions to ask were firstly - whether the research findings were correct? Because, if they were then the second question to ask was – is whether the treatment and the whole treatment strategy worked or was effective?

The first question was asked but never really was disputed. There never really was an opportunity to ask the second question. So much money had been committed, there were government and ministerial reputations to maintain, a Special Health Authority in the name of the National Treatment Agency and NHS and voluntary sector providers' reputations to maintain.

No one in the Drugs Treatment caravan was going to be stupid enough to question whether the initial premise was correct. Everyone was knee deep in money that had never been there before.

So instead, we then proceeded along a 10 year strategy of stating 'more treatment, better treatment, fairer treatment'. An entire monitoring system was established to prove the strategy was working, based on outcomes that mattered little in relation to what a drug user wanted or needed. The argument shifted to the wider drug use and finally just as patience and outcomes were threadbare thin, the new approach to getting people out of treatment and into recovery, whether they were capable of recovery or not – everybody was aboard the new bandwagon, so users needed to get their arses into gear because this was the Big Society.

The last 12 years have been what I would describe as policy driven evidence driving treatment. You like to think that it is an evidence base that drives policy and treatment. It is a very important and quite frightening difference.

One of the very significant issues that came out of this was that there appeared to be a key group of drug users who were responsible for a high level of crime in some areas. Once this evidence was clear then some very constructive and effective work could be done.

Unfortunately by then, every drug user had been labelled as a criminal. The treatment services had had an influx of offenders who also took drugs as opposed to serious drug users whose criminality was to feed a habit. For offenders who took drugs the treatment options and non-custodial sentences offered opportunities too good to turn down and for some it offered them additional free drugs through substitute prescribing.

This is the kind of thing that happens when you take a broad sweep approach.

What we know about alcohol is actually quite a lot. We have very clear statistical information on how much people drink, the numbers at risk and the numbers with serious problems. We know the incidence of alcohol-related accidents, alcohol-related NHS bed occupancy, child abuse, domestic violence, drink driving and other alcohol-related violence.

We know about alcohol consumption, types of consumption by products, regional variations and trends, use by age. We know how many licensed premises there are in the UK and where they all are.

We know how alcohol affects the body and the brain.

We know what type of interventions work and for whom to a pretty good degree.

Where it becomes blurred is:

• The fact that the health messages that we have do not really help those who are drinking too much.

- The general population do not really understand how harmful alcohol as a drug is to the body, especially because it is a legal drug.
- That some groups of the population are more susceptible to alcohol-related harm and again the general population need to understand why that is the case.
- That overcoming a serious alcohol problem is a relapsing condition. Most people take many attempts to reach abstinence or to change their behaviour. However the message and expectation of recovery makes relapse seen continuously as a failure.

Some of the research published over the last ten to fifteen years about consumption rates is contradictory and confusing – for example, drinking a glass of red wine is good for you; not drinking for three days is good for you; bingeing (over four units in one session) is bad.

What we need is a review of existing research and findings by a group of independent researchers to give us a balanced overall analysis of what the research tells us. We can then place that against what we know from the facts and figures. We can then analyse the treatment outcomes against milestone research of treatment such as Project MATCH.

Project MATCH began in 1989 in the United States and was sponsored by the National Institute on Alcohol Abuse and Alcoholism (NIAAA). The project was an 8-year, multi-site, $27-million investigation that studied which types of alcoholics respond best to which forms of treatment. MATCH studied whether treatment should be uniform or assigned to patients based on specific needs and characteristics. The programs were administered by psychotherapists and, although twelve-step methods were incorporated into the therapy, actual AA meetings were not included.

Three types of treatment were investigated:

Cognitive Behavioural Coping Skills Therapy, focusing on correcting poor self-esteem and distorted, negative, and self-defeating thinking.

Motivational Enhancement Therapy, which helps clients to become aware of and build on personal strengths that can help improve readiness to quit.

Twelve-Step Facilitation Therapy administered as an independent treatment designed to familiarize patients with the AA philosophy and to encourage participation.

The study concluded that patient-treatment matching is not necessary in alcoholism treatment because the three techniques are equal in effectiveness.

What is less reported is that there was a wide discrepancy in treatment outcomes from different sites of the same programme, which indicates that there are significant other factors influencing outcomes such as the individual seeking support.

Finally as part of a research strategy we can then commission the research that is still needed.

Asking the right questions

In this debate we probably do need to ask the question whether we want to keep alcohol as our legal drug? Banning alcohol would be a major issue and after the experience of Prohibition in the USA, it would be a very high risk strategy. The author would be very much against such a move but it does need to be asked because of the following:

At the moment we have an unofficial body (the Independent Scientific Committee on Drugs) classifying alcohol as the third most dangerous drug, with over twenty banned drugs classified below it (this is the committee Professor David Nutt established after resigning as Chair of the ACMD, which was the official government Body for the classification of drugs.) We have Royal Colleges calling for major price increases and trade restrictions and warning us of disastrous health consequences and drinking epidemics. All this happens, while the government earns £14 billion in tax and duty and as a response tells us about sensible drinking limits and urging us all to drink responsibly.

The gap between the two is a chasm and people are genuinely confused. There is no credibility for any health message with these contradictions.

Perhaps the real root of the whole problem lies between the Treasury and Public and National Health.

We need to ask the obvious questions about alcohol because at the moment they blame the alcohol producers and the retail trade. They point the finger at the 8 million who drink over recommended safe limits. When it comes to the odd 1.5 million with a serious alcohol misuse problem, then they are all personally weak and responsible for their own downfall.

There is not a hint that there is something terribly wrong structurally.

Therefore, by having a rational debate and asking the question – do we want to keep alcohol legal and available to us then we do have a credible base on which to frame our future. By asking this basic question, we are making a choice as a society. My guess is that we would choose to continue with having alcohol as a legal substance.

I strongly believe that the first outcome of this 'national decision' would be to highlight this structural problem between the Treasury and Public Health. It should put to an end the long running arguments between Public and National Health officials and lobbyists and the wider 'alcohol industry' and finally silence the self-appointed moralists.

Such an outcome would force the two antagonists to work within a broad agreement of what needs to be done to reduce the harm. This should not require statutes or law changes. It might involve a few sackings but that would be no bad thing to my mind.

What would be in this broad agreement? What information and research do we need to be clear about who are the vulnerable groups at risk in society? How do we want to develop as a society with our drinking in the future? Presumably in a way which enhances the enjoyment and leisure aspects whilst reducing the alcohol-related violence and disorder? How do we encourage our population to drink in less harmful ways to their health?

- Once we know who these groups are then how are we to help them? What tools and information and practical support can they be given?
- What does our public health information on alcohol need to contain and where should it be available?
- Whose job is it to deliver these messages once we know what is needed and where?
- What do our retail outlets need to look like in the wake of this new approach to alcohol and drinking?
- What do we need to teach our young people and young adults?
- What terminology do we need to have to effectively help people in the future and what do we need to abandon?
- What treatment interventions do we need to have in place across every health and local authority?
- What medical services do we need to have in place to back up these treatment interventions?

Understanding our collective drinking history

We need to come to understand our current drinking behaviour and the drinking culture that we have inherited. We need to understand the drivers for our drinking culture. The run through of the history of interventions in this book demonstrate how different interventions greatly influence drinking patterns and types of drinking, from government to war to economics to religion.

Yet most importantly, we need to appreciate and understand that beyond all these interventions is our desire, passion and need to drink intoxicating beverages, sometimes despite the political climate and influences.

To consider drinking at the turn of the twentieth century compared with the end of the same century, we are told the overall level of drinking had returned to the same as it was in 1900 but with huge changes over the intervening ninety nine years.

This is hardly surprising with two World Wars, Spanish Flu, the Great Depression, rationing followed by massive deregulation and alcohol becoming available everywhere.

It would seem from reading history, every century is the same, with some centuries clearly being more soaked in alcohol than others. There is no denying though that drinking alcohol is a permanent feature in any given decade and century.

We have a heavy drinking culture, where intoxication and getting drunk is the expected 'norm'.

However, within this 'norm' are an enormous range of different attitudes and beliefs – throughout history there are religious groups who do not drink – sometimes dominant and sometimes not. At times it was safer to drink beer and spirits than water.

Britain never really had a great history as a wine drinking nation (until the last few decades). The Romans bought the vine to the UK for cultivation and wine to drink but it was the drinking of ale (beer) and mead that was popular for centuries and latterly - in the last 1,000 years - spirits.

This pattern of drinking is very similar to the rest of northern Europe, but with an island mentality. It is significantly different to southern Europe. It is within this culture and climate that drinking behaviour was established. In today's terminology, it would be considered bingeing. Our Norsemen, Britons, Scots, Irish and Saxons would consider it as normal male drinking – an essential part of life and celebration, of drinking to the gods, of being a man and a warrior or a farmer or a sailor, being at one with and defying the natural forces. I do not believe that anyone watched their units when drinking in their great halls and talking about Valhalla.

This may sound trite but it is part of our cultural history and it has continued throughout history with every wave of newcomer to the shores of Britain. Europe brought us lager, the peoples of the West Indies bought us rum, the French and Italians wine again.

Whatever anyone brought to these islands we have imbibed with gusto and greed and passion. I really do not think it is a type of drink that matters – it is THE drink. The industry does a fantastic job promoting and advertising their products and encouraging us to drink but even without too much promotion the majority of the people of this island will drink and have always drunk to excess.

Is it learnt or in the DNA or am I wrong? Every time I ask this question, I can think of twenty people who do not drink much and I can think of twenty others who drink a lot and I can think of a handful who have developed significant problems (and that is outside of my work).

The human desire to take something into our body that affects our perception of the world; that affects our emotions and influences our insight has been strong from when our first ancestors squeezed into dark caves to paint on the rock walls through to the present day.

A vast library has been written on this subject about different drugs through many and varied cultures. Alcohol is no different, it is a drug and it has all these effects on the working of the human brain. This fact should never be forgotten in all this debate. The truth of the matter is that it is completely ignored in our Public Health approach.

Somewhere in this whole debate we have to accept our history if we are to move forward.

Pricing Revisited

There is now a plan to bring in a minimum price for a unit of alcohol. It is a cornerstone of the new government Alcohol Strategy. The traditional argument has been that increasing the price of a drink will reduce the overall demand for drinks. This is without doubt true when it is about overall levels of consumption.

Increasing the price of alcohol by introducing a minimum price or linking the price to strength will have an immediate impact on anyone who has limited or low income, who can 'take it or leave it', or who has a family. Social drinkers may have one less of a night.

Such a pricing policy will reduce overall demand because it will impact on the majority of people. It will be unpopular because it is affecting all the wrong people and it will be a failure because it will not target those who need to be targeted.

Even worse, anyone who has a significant alcohol problem or dependency is highly unlikely to be able to reduce their alcohol intake based purely on price. To afford the same level of beverages at an increased overall price then money will need to be diverted from some other form of spend. They will eat less food, spend less on their children, heating or rent. Minimum pricing or unit pricing will simply make the problem worse for those experiencing the worst problems.

This approach is particularly upsetting from an economic point of view because we were taught even at O-level economics that throughout history when the price of bread increased people sometimes bought more bread because it meant they could no longer afford to eat both bread and some meat, so that instead they could eat more bread and no meat.

The other by-product of this increased pricing strategy is the tipping point where you can guarantee increased crime—shoplifting, illegal home brewing, organised illegal brewing and smuggling.

The example in relation to cigarettes is there for all to see. The continual price increases has led to importation of cigarettes on a massive scale. Cigarettes retailing at £1.50 in the Ukraine find their way to the UK to be sold on the street and undercover. An articulated lorry load of cigarettes would make the importer a millionaire overnight while the government loses an awfully large sum of lost duty and tax. At least these imports are authorised and inspected cigarettes. The other aspect of this pricing campaign has been to encourage the manufacture of counterfeit cigarettes.

Counterfeit cigarettes are truly scary – poor standards, no regulation, and dangerous components with massive health risks.

It is the same for alcohol – the production of illegal alcohol is a growing and thriving business around the world and there is evidence that this is happening in the UK.

This is the price we all pay when our 'health tsars' and lobbyists are allowed to push regulation and pricing to limits where there is no research nor understanding of human beings and economic markets.

Unintended consequences are always a risk to any change in policy. However, most of what we are discussing here are not unintended consequences because the research and market knowledge is there for all to see.

Suffice to say, pricing needs to always be carefully considered but as a tool for restraining trade and consumption it is a lazy and ineffective option.

A new approach to Alcohol Information and Awareness

We need to have an alcohol awareness and information strategy that has both a preventative and harm reduction approach to drinking and associated risk behaviour.

You might have guessed it by now but implicit in any new approach to alcohol information and awareness should be without the use of units of alcohol. I have laid out very clearly why units of alcohol are not only misleading but wrong in the way they are presented. Worse still, the whole 'units of alcohol' message is not that well understood and is largely ignored because of circumstance.

A unit of alcohol may be measurable to a standard drink but look at any description of twenty standard drinks in a pub and the units vary on almost every single one and that is where we are measuring, unlike at home, parties, barbecues, holidays and social gatherings.

For me the use of units is like becoming a member of a special group or an exclusive club. Currently everything available to support alcohol harm reduction is referenced by units of alcohol. It is a bit like you need to wear a tie to enter a members club, or no trainers at a night club, or having the right connections or schooling to enter Parliament.

Normal everyday behaviour and thinking becomes subservient to trying to calculate your unit intake. It really is nonsense.

Alcohol Harm Reduction is about changing behaviour and the way we drink, which then influences the amount we drink. Talking about quantity on its own becomes meaningless and unhelpful. Making a cake requires a quantity of flour, milk and butter – that does not tell you how to make a cake.

A new approach to Alcohol Information and Awareness should be run by the drinks industry and the licensed trade, in partnership with Public Health. The Information and Awareness needs to happen in the pubs and clubs, in the supermarkets and all licensed retail outlets. Of course it still needs to be available in GP surgeries and places like libraries. It needs to be where those who are drinking can have access to it.

The partnerships with local authorities, with Health and Social Care Agencies, with the Police and Probation Service still need to happen.

Information should be available in every licensed premise. It should be a requirement as part of a licence. The information needs to be easily seen, giving simple facts and guidance on drinking effects and risk, together with contact details on where to obtain advice and help (and one of the cheapest ways in a public house is to put it on the beer mats).

The information that is available to the people of the UK should be just that – information. Not messages but easy-to-understand information. Information that enables each and every one of us to risk assess for ourselves and to understand what happens to us as we drink and how our cognitive processes are affected.

To make this a reality, then in the short term (two or three years) at least £1 billion needs to be diverted from the Treasury into this Alcohol Awareness and Information Strategy. Alternatively, the income could just stay within the drinks industry and be spent directly by them, with this spend being accountable to the public.

It also needs to be done with humour and laughter, because that is how we remember and how we break down barriers. Some of the most memorable advertising campaigns for drinks involve humour. Humour is an essential vehicle for learning and remembering.

We are working with behaviour change remember, and humour is a key factor in how we see and influence behaviour change. Otherwise we will be in danger of just repeating current approaches of telling people how to behave and how to think.

We also need to move away from being told to be sensible and responsible. Do not remove fun and laughter – what we are trying to do is to reduce harm, reduce consumption whilst maintaining (or increasing) happiness and fun. Our approach has to mirror what we are trying to achieve. It again sounds simple and trite but that is the essence of what we need to create. Somewhere in this we are of course trying to persuade people to be responsible in their own outcome behaviour – not being abusive or violent, unnecessarily noisy or angry.

Unfortunately, some people are abusive and violent, noisy and angry and alcohol merely acts as an accelerant or lubricant for this behaviour. This is where we have to create an environment where peers and family take the lead in curbing some individuals' excesses. I return you to the example of the wedding where a number of men avoid the whiskey and brandy because that is when the fists come up.

Over time and painful experience of broken and bloodied noses, family schisms and arrests, men (and some women) have learnt to curb their drinking or curb their tongue when drinking. Part of this approach has to be to try to encourage this to happen faster and across all our communities.

This is not just about drinking culture and behaviour. It forms part of a wider culture change to reduce violence and disrespect to one another and to produce better tolerance and civility.

Brief Interventions and Practical Support

The second part of this book was all about explaining that reducing harmful drinking and overcoming a significant drinking problem is pretty simple and straight forward. It is not rocket science. The interventions that I am promoting here are simply about two or three hour to two hour sessions looking at how to reduce your drinking and tactics for tackling/addressing some of the problems that are causing difficulties.

No one needs a label of seeing a counsellor, or being a problem drinker. You are simply spending two or three sessions to look at your patterns of drinking, why they are the way they are and how to make some changes. It is something normal to do like going to the dentist or doctor.

It will not work for everyone but it will make a difference for an awful lot of people.

I would argue that there needs to be a further diversion of £0.5 billion into primary health care specifically ring fenced for alcohol-related problems for a couple of years. This would ensure that up to three Brief Intervention sessions would be available to any person through their GP.

This would have a massive impact on our drinking.

Treatment Interventions

Finally, a further diversion of £0.5 billion needs to go into alcohol treatment. Every local authority needs to have a specialist alcohol treatment service offering crisis intervention with residential or community detoxification, stabilisation services, brief interventions, a treatment programme of groups designed to teach cutting down or stopping, relapse prevention, abstinence and controlled drinking programmes.

It needs to openly support and advertise AA, Al Anon and AL Ateen Groups. The programme needs to link up with housing and social services, probation and health. These services need to be on a level of provision with existing drug services.

It is a lot of money but it does not need to be year on year for the next ten years. However, it certainly will require a massive effort if this nation is to change. We need to accept that the actual costs associated with the current levels of drinking will reduce in the long term if something like this is done now.

Only in this way will we manage to target a reduction in alcohol-related harm across the general population and a permanent reduction from Brief Interventions and Treatment.

To back all of this up, then we need to see the following happen:

Revisiting our Licensing Requirements

There needs to be a properly researched review on the Licensing Act. The classic question would be - has the new extended hours worked in terms of being popular? Has alcohol-related violence and disorder increased or decreased?

However, underneath this obvious question may well be that extended hours are a good thing but we never educated the people to live with extended hours. All we did was extend the hours to enable everyone to spend longer behaving in the same way as we did with limited hours. I heard Ministers suggesting that we could have continental drinking in the UK.

The result we seem to have ended up with is that we drink underneath heaters, in a roped off area outside of a licensed premises, drinking a £4 bottle of lager. Parallel with this was the passing of by–laws which banned public drinking in any other areas. This ensured that the homeless street drinker was not allowed in the same vicinity.

How do we decide how many licensed premises we should have in any one area and who can decide? Local people and their authorities surely need to be given the freedom to determine their own level of desired licensed premises in their locality taking into account local requirements and dynamics.

The drunken chaos of our city centres at night is not acceptable yet as a nation we do accept it. Filming it has become prime time. Watching people falling over, fighting and being sick can be seen on numerous TV channels – throw in plenty of swearing, wobbling stomachs, fat white bums falling out of trousers and TV blurred (obscured) tits and faces and to add to the horror of the reality we have hit TV shows.

This armchair voyeurism has a much more serious and sinister side – sexual assault and rape, stranger violence, attack to property and danger to emergency services across the Police and NHS.

Any new approach to our drinking behaviour and culture needs something to change.

It should no longer be acceptable for a pub or nightclub to serve someone until they are intoxicated and then simply eject them onto the streets.

Perhaps a more effective arrangement to encourage licensed establishments to operate within the law would be to have them hold their customers on their premises until they are sober or can be accompanied home. They might then try to manage that descent into intoxication in a very different manner.

It has to be acknowledged that there is a pretty large gap between being merry and drunk and falling down drunk, unable to speak and stand, pissing themselves, which appears to be increasingly standard behaviour for many. This has required a lot of drinking and the supply to create that level of intoxication has been sanctioned within a venue. The law as it stands has been clearly violated and the response of that premise is usually to get them off the premises.

In a nutshell, when a venue allows someone to become drunk (it is still illegal to serve alcohol to someone who is intoxicated) then they can deal with the consequences or acknowledge that they had broken existing laws and face the legal consequences. This does not require new laws, just the upholding of existing ones. The police should not have to – they have more important work to do.

There is a clear choice here – uphold and enforce the law or change it. Do not just ignore it and flaunt it and then dump the consequences onto someone else. If the venue will not take responsibility then the local authority and the police can. They have the power to close down premises for periods of time. I am not advocating this course of action – what I am saying is that ignoring it or colluding with it will only make the behaviour worse. It all needs careful unpicking.

As was proposed earlier, every licensed premise needs to have information and contact details in the establishment as part of their license.

What the alcohol producers and retailers need to do

Many commentators I have spoken to in the last five years consider many of the larger companies who produce alcoholic beverages to be arrogant and highly reluctant to manage significant change to their industry; high on rhetoric and very slick in their PR approach. This is a view borne out by their experiences in trying to work with them.

Indeed, some commentators would be more vociferous in their criticism. My own view, for what it is worth, is that they would probably take a very different approach if the wider political and social commentary involved the general population and not just the current small band that is ranged against them. To try to bring these divides closer together there are some very quick and effective actions the 'industry' could take to show their commitment to some honest and constructive change:

- To bring in straight away, a limit on the size of a bottle or can of lagers, beers and ciders over 6 per cent down to 33 cl.
- This could then be followed by a review of whether we need to have any beers, lagers and cider over a certain percentage (such as 6 per cent). What is the market for these

drinks? Are most of these products bought mainly by those with serious alcohol problems? If this is the case then there should be general agreement that they should be removed but not until we have the facts to hand rather than anecdotal evidence.

• The wider drinks industry could make funding available for the research that is required.

• Stop sponsoring sport. The industry will argue that Budweisers' new sponsorship arrangement with the FA Cup highly promotes the Drinkaware Trust work. Although going in the right direction, perhaps the future could be the FA Cup sponsored by Drinkaware. The level of alcohol-related harm in the UK should warrant a consensus that drinks companies do not need to associate themselves with sport.

• To demonstrate that they are a responsible industry. They say that they are and some parts of the producers and retailers are, but some parts are not and they need to be brought up to the standard of those who are responsible or closed down. The drink aware campaigns are a start but licensed premises need to be better maintained and managed.

The industry has to start to acknowledge in a significant way that its products can be dangerous, that alcohol does cause social and physical harm. The tobacco industry has acknowledged that its products are harmful and the work is on to produce not only less harmful smoking products but to find alternatives at getting nicotine into the body. The tobacco industry is still getting kicked and the time is hopefully approaching where a dialogue and partnership will be formed that really creates effective harm reduction for smokers. But with alcohol there is still arrogance by some in the alcohol industry that does not accept that change needs to happen in a more constructive way.

A National Training Strategy

There needs to be a National Training Strategy for all Public Health and Social Care staff on alcohol and drinking, so that everyone has access to basic information and advice from a professional.

Alcohol and Crime and Disorder

The current link between alcohol and crime is there for all to see. It is the most obvious link in today's society and there should be no pretense.

It is a factor in 50 per cent of stranger violence and domestic violence (and 86 per cent of murders), it is strongly linked to disorder and antisocial behaviour, especially in city centres. Drink driving is an offence. Alcohol use and problematic drinking is acknowledged as a factor for many who commit shoplifting, burglary, robbery, criminal damage and arson. Alcohol misuse is a factor in domestic violence and child abuse.

These links and facts are known. They are not made up. Anyone who works in government, the Home Office, Ministry of Justice, Criminal Justice Policy, courts, police and the probation service know about these facts and they choose in reality to do very little about it.

This is not acceptable. It is not acceptable to have the level of domestic violence that we have in this country, nor stranger violence, nor city centre disorder. It is a national issue and a personal issue. It is an issue that everyone needs to address. Collectively, we should be ashamed that so much domestic violence is allowed to take place.

Let us pause there for one moment. This unacceptable level of violence is caused mostly by men. Their attitudes, aggression and violence appears born from cultural beliefs and values. The

British appear to often associate drinking with being aggressive and violent, often verbally, and as their drinking descends into drunkenness then physical aggression and violence. Drinking also provides the excuse for violence – 'it was the drink! He is not like that when he has not been drinking'.

The problem is that sober, merry or drunk, it was the person who glassed or punched the other person. This book argues for a re-evaluation of our culture and what environmental, social, economic, political and personal values create these attitudes, these behaviours, and this mind set.

The government's New Alcohol Strategy does not address any of this. Prime Minister Cameron points out that it is jolly serious and has to stop and he does not mind being unpopular with his measures to counter this. His rhetoric is one thing, the reality another. He is basing the whole strategy on pricing bad behaviour out of existence.

He believes that by introducing a minimum price per unit of alcohol, this will change the behaviour of all these people. Commentators in Cameron's own cabinet described the idea of minimum pricing to tackle binge drinking as absurd. Need more be said here?

Well actually, yes it does. The government also introduced the idea of tackling pre-loading. I read this idea of pre-loading with intrigue. It was what I thought you did with a washing machine in order to tackle difficult stains. The minimum pricing would stop individuals buying their drinks in supermarkets and corner shops and drinking them before they went out, or pre-loading their evening.

For me, it represents cowardice politics – strong words and what looks like tough and effective action with little or no impact, no attempt to grapple with the underlying issues and trying to keep everyone vaguely on board (the drink and retail industry, the police, the NHS and the medical lobby).

Try and address the fundamental issues and it is an opportunity to massively reduce crime and to make the UK a better place to live in.

Those who commit these alcohol-related offences end up in our criminal justice system at enormous cost to the nation.

Prisons are virtually full of individuals who have an alcohol, drug or mental health problem. Around 50 per cent will have experienced homelessness or very temporary accommodation. Drinking goes virtually hand in hand with this vicious cycle. The prison service needs to be systematically geared up to support these profiles. At the moment, anyone who leaves prison with an alcohol (or drug) problem and manages to cope with their circumstances and all the demands placed on them and *not* return to old drinking or drug using ways is an amazing person.

Probation and the Courts need to be geared up to ensure that many of those before them are supported through the programmes proposed rather than through the current system. These programmes need to be meaningful, with training and learning opportunities, apprenticeships, decent housing support, budgeting and basic coping skills. They need to be able to avoid their old 'friends' (their drinking and drug using network) and they need treatment support that is safe and worthwhile (and dare I say it – enjoyable).

What do we know about what we need to do? Let us take a look at one aspect of alcohol-related crime – drink driving.

Drink Driving

Drink driving is an interesting issue because there is so much that can be done. Drink drive offenders fall between those who knowingly and intentionally break the law in the full knowledge that they are unlikely to ever be caught and those who think that they have not drunk enough to be over the legal limit.

The obvious answer is to have more systematic testing by the police but their resources are stretched, so such an approach needs to be seen as a priority by the police authority. In turn the police need to be supported by the government. In France it is law for every car to have a breathalyser kit (along with luminous jackets, a first aid kit and a breakdown triangle). This would be a good thing to introduce into the UK. It has the message of self-responsibility for some aspects of health and safety and reducing risk. No bad thing at all. Licensed premises can provide free cab numbers, free or cheap soft drinks for delegated drivers and even a responsibility to not serve customers who have cars in the car park.

Friends and family should see they have the moral responsibility and courage to try to persuade the driver not to drink. That is where the decision making happens and if the driver insists on drinking then each passenger has a decision to make for themselves. It is not down to a police officer or a politician. It is where the individual sand in the line is drawn for each and every one of us.

It is a fact that many people on drink driving courses as a result of conviction do not understand units of alcohol and the strengths of different drinks and drink driving limits. As we know drinking three units of alcohol stops us bingeing in terms of official definition but three units will have taken some people into having over 50 milligrams of alcohol in their bloodstream. So that would seem to indicate that the messages are not working.

So if we are to make inroads at reducing drink driving we have to increase the risk of getting caught, create an environment where third parties can put pressure on a potential drink driver to desist and finally we have to equip people with the knowledge and the facts. That even one or two drinks will slow your reaction, giving you much better odds at running over someone who steps out in front of you. You are not a better driver with drink in you. You are drinking a drug. This drug will not only slow your reactions but will affect your judgement and you will be a risk taker.

We need messages that are clear that if you are driving do not drink or if you have to then just one drink, not two or three, but one. The main message is do not drink, get a taxi, walk or take it in turns.

Finally for someone who is caught and has broken the law, then sentences need to reflect the seriousness of the risk taken - bans for driving need to be for a minimum of three years for a first offence no matter what the level of intoxication. A second offence needs to carry a ban for ten years. The tool for destruction has then been removed, fines could still be considered but the emphasis is on taking away someone's legal ability to go out and commit an offence that could maim or kill. In the case of prison, we already have appropriate sentencing for someone who has caused injury or death.

Reducing drink driving cannot happen with just one wave of a wand. It requires a systematic and concerted approach which needs to overlap across a range of measures. This is the same for most other criminal justice issues. We have to challenge the behaviour and we have to look at the context of the behaviour and understand how to change it.

Domestic violence, stranger violence, city centre fighting and disorder all need to be approached in the same way as drink driving. The behaviour needs to be made unacceptable by all parties, information needs to be available, venues need to understand their responsibilities and what the law states in terms of serving policy and how they manage intoxicated customers. It all needs to be concerted and concentrated.

Again, offenders need to be appropriately worked with and sentenced where the level of violence warrants it.

We know that anger management and alcohol groups work, when they are factual and designed to assist the offender rather than being seen as part of a punishment. When this behaviour is placed against a changing background attitude then this work becomes easier and more effective.

The criminal justice agencies of the courts, probation and prison simply have to start to make alcohol-related offending a priority. This needs to be directed by government and money needs to be spent on both training the staff and introducing programmes and content that will assist the alcohol-related offender.

Brief Interventions, education, group work (anger management, stopping drinking and reducing drinking groups) and relapse prevention work will have an impact on reducing re-offending through drinking. It will however only be effective if it is embraced as a meaningful programme rather than the usual tough talking strategy with little money or resources to back it up. It has to be real (as was described previously).

So how can you have an alcohol strategy without considering Class, Inequality and Poverty?

To answer the question, this book has clearly made the case that you cannot (and should not).

Poverty is a much misunderstood term these days. Whenever poverty is discussed it seems to be derailed in the UK. How can anyone suggest that they are living in poverty when they have a satellite dish and people still drink and smoke? The whole debate about inequalities of wealth and diet and substance use is a minefield.

However, in the UK, health related diseases such as diabetes and heart disease, who is at risk and how they are treated are very clearly related to issues of wealth inequality. It is a fact that there is huge wealth inequality in the UK. The latest Alcohol Strategy (and the Drug Strategy) does not reference this fact in any way. How we behave as consumers and how our health is, are huge and significant factors in how we drink, eat, live (and smoke and use drugs) in relation to our wealth or lack of it. Why then is this ignored if any strategy is going to be effective?

The trouble for alcohol is that it is treated as if it is an entity in itself. It is described as a substance and everything from beer to lager to wine to spirits to liqueurs is described as alcohol in most of the literature and research (which indeed they are) which tends to alienate the substance – alcohol, from the products. It has its own government strategy (like drugs) and it is quantified in measurements of units. There is not one reference to health inequalities.

The added trouble for alcohol and its related problems is that it is always someone else who is the problem. Theresa May, the Home Secretary, when she could answer how much she drank in a week, pointed out that it was not her who went around causing mayhem in the city centre at weekends. Everyone else's drinking behaviour is the problem.

The next problem for alcohol is that the 10 per cent of people with 80 per cent of the alcohol-related health problems happens to be the poorest. Why is such a hugely significant dynamic not even worthy of a comment or a reference?

Furthermore, if drinking (and drug use) touches the more privileged classes then in it is an individual tragedy or a personal weakness. For the people that Theresa May refers to they are a disgrace and need to be controlled and punished. The Home Secretary appears to have the view these pre-loaders are just out to cause trouble. The fact that you may not have much disposable income and want to enjoy a drink as much as anyone else but cannot afford pub and club prices is ignored. How to try to combat the behaviour that is unacceptable has to be tackled and addressed structurally, not with a price increase for god's sake.

We know that alcohol consumption measured by units is a convenient public health message that lumps the poor, the well off and the rich together when not only their income but their work (or lack of it), their housing, their diet and as a consequence their health and their children's health and opportunities is completely different.

The Coalition government want people not to pre-load before they go out. Their approach is to raise the unit price and stop cheap deals. It is blatantly targeting the poorer person who can only afford to buy cheap drinks.

This is why we have an alcohol strategy and a drug strategy, rather than a wealth inequality strategy which addresses health inequalities, poor diet, and substance misuse and its disproportionate impact on the poorest.

So any future thinking and practical approach to our drinking has to take these factors into account, otherwise it is a worthless and redundant exercise. When health policies lead to increased crime and make no headway into parts of our society then it is not only failing but contributing to our overall decline. The market for illegally imported alcohol and even the illicit production of alcoholic drinks (counterfeiting) is on the increase. No one should be surprised.

Nature abhors a vacuum – there are tipping points throughout nature and history when enough is enough and the unintended consequences of planned action far outweigh the intended beneficial outcomes.

None of the above requires additional funding through the Public Purse. This is a re-distribution of income from the sale and duty on alcohol into expenditure on alcohol-related harm, ill health and prevention. Of course this will require savings on areas of spending that the alcohol tax and duty was spent on.

This book calls for such a radical overhaul because without it, this country and its people will continue to suffer alcohol-related ill health and violence and disorder.

A Glass Half Full

APPENDIX 1

Drink Diary

Purpose – the idea of you having a drink diary is for you to keep a personal record of drinking, how much and why, who with and what it costs. This then helps you look at not only the amount but patterns of your drinking behaviour.

You can then overlap this with what is going on elsewhere in your life and to begin to understand the role and impact your drinking has.

Week Number............

Day of the week	What time did you start drinking?	The number of hours you were drinking?	Where were you drinking?
Monday			
Tuesday			
Wednesday			
Thursday			
Friday			
Saturday			
Sunday			

Who were you drinking with?	What did you drink and how much?	How much did you spend?	Write a little commentary – how you were feeling, any reasons for drinking. Did you mix drink with any other drugs?

Notes/comments on the whole week

A Glass Half Full

APPENDIX 2

AUDIT TOOL

The Alcohol Use Disorders Identification Test (AUDIT) was developed by the World Health Organization in 1982 as a simple way to screen and identify people who are at risk of developing alcohol problems.

The AUDIT test focuses on identifying the preliminary signs of hazardous drinking and mild dependence. It is used to detect alcohol problems experienced within the last year. It is one of the most accurate alcohol screening tests available, rated 92 per cent effective in detecting hazardous or harmful drinking.

The test contains 10 multiple choice questions on the amount and frequency of alcohol consumption, drinking behaviour and alcohol-related problems or reactions. On average it should take two minutes to complete.

The answers are scored on a point system, with different scores indicating different actions to be taken.

Scores:	0	1	2	3	4	Your score
How often do you have a drink containing alcohol?	Never	Monthly or less	2-4 times per month	2-3 times per week	4+ times per week	
How many units of alcohol do you drink on a typical day when you are drinking?	1-2	3-4	5-6	7-8	10+	
How often have you had 6 or more units if female, or 8 or more if male, on a single occasion in the last year?	Never	Less than monthly	Monthly	Weekly	Daily or almost daily	
How often during the last year have you found that you were not able to stop drinking once you had started?	Never	Less than monthly	Monthly	Weekly	Daily or almost daily	
How often during the last year have you found that you were not able to stop drinking once you had started?	Never	Less than monthly	Monthly	Weekly	Daily or almost daily	
How often during the last year have you failed to do what was normally expected from you because of your drinking?	Never	Less than monthly	Monthly	Weekly	Daily or almost daily	

Scores:	0	1	2	3	4	Your score
How often during the last year have you needed an alcoholic drink in the morning to get yourself going after a heavy drinking session?	Never	Less than monthly	Monthly	Weekly	Daily or almost daily	
How often during the last year have you had a feeling of guilt or remorse after drinking?	Never	Less than monthly	Monthly	Weekly	Daily or almost daily	
How often during the last year have you been unable to remember what happened the night before because you had been drinking?	Never	Less than monthly	Monthly	Weekly	Daily or almost daily	
Have you or somebody else been injured as a result of your drinking?	No		Yes, but not in the last year		Yes, during the last year	
Has a relative or friend, doctor or other health worker been concerned about your drinking or suggested that you cut down?	No		Yes, but not in the last year		Yes, during the last year	

Scoring: 0-7 lower risk, 8-15 increasing risk, 16-19 higher risk, 20+ possible dependence

Your score _____

Acknowledgements

This book has been thirty years in the writing. What has been written owes inspiration from a myriad of men and woman, who I have been lucky to meet and to work with. As I said at the beginning of this book, those men and woman who have overcome their personal battles, addictions or problems have my utmost respect and admiration.

Without doubt, members of the New Directions in the Study of alcohol Group (NDSAG) informed and challenged me the most. The NDSAG are a group of people with no allegiances, no exclusivity, no sponsors and no public or private funding. Thank you one and all.

My thanks go to Christopher Snowdon for helping me get this published and for his open and honest feedback. Aidan Gray for his unfailing support, insight and thinking and of course his sense of humour. Also for his cover design and his experience of photographing a pint in a pub as he was drinking it – he made it sound like going on a date! He made me think and he gave me confidence in what I was writing. Trevor McCarthy has done the same over the years. Never short of an opinion but always able to provide a different insight. On many an occasion I could telephone either of them and they would listen to me ranting of vice versa. I would also like to thank Claire Brown the editor of Drink and Drug News, who read my first ever draft of this book and made some very helpful comments which encouraged me to continue.

Finally, thank you Teresa, for being you (my best friend and my soul mate), giving me your love and the space to finally sit and write this, to read the drafts and believe in me.

About the Author

Andy founded and ran an alcohol charity (Rugby House in 1986 through to December 2008). Before that he worked in an alcohol charity (ARP) for 4 years. During his Social Work training, he completed a placement at an alcohol treatment unit at Warwick Hospital and in his words 'became addicted to the world of alcohol' from there. He has a Ba in Psychology and a Masters in Social Policy on alcohol as well as a Social Work Qualification (but never has been a social worker).

In relation to alcohol, he likes a few drinks (there go us all by the grace of Gaia).

His heroes and heroines are the men and women who have climbed out of their own personal hell holes and overcome their alcohol and drug dependencies. His anti-hero's and heroines are all the men and women in government and in the government departments who have denied, ignored or colluded with never trying to address the problem over the last 30 years, when they were in a position to do so. They know who they are!

Lightning Source UK Ltd.
Milton Keynes UK
UKOW042151270313

208309UK00001B/36/P